MW01520202

A List of the General and Field-officers, as They Rank in the Army. Of the Officers of the Several Regiments ... Complete to September, 1758. To Which is now Added, the Succession of Colonels

J. O. Travers

By PERMISSION of the RIGHT HONOURABLE

The SECRETARY at WAR.

A

LIST

OF THE

GENERAL and FIELD-OFFICERS,

As they Rank in the ARMY.

Of the OFFICERS,

IN THE

SEVERAL REGIMENTS

OF

HORSE, DRAGOONS, and FOOT,

ON THE

BRITISH and IRISH ESTABLISHMENTS:

WITH

The Dates of their COMMISSIONS, as they Rank in each CORPS, and as they Rank in the ARMY.

The Royal REGIMENT of ARTILLERY, IRISH ARTILLERY, ENGINEERS, the MARINES, and INDEPENDENT COMPANIES.

GOVERNORS, LIEUTENANT-GOVERNORS, of His Majesty's GARRISONS at Home and Abroad, with their ALLOWANCES, and the OFFICERS on HALF PAY, &c. Complete to *SEPTEMBER*, 1758.

To which is now added,

The SUCCESSION of COLONELS.

LONDON:

Printed for J. MILLAN, opposite the *Admiralty-Office*.

[Price 3*s*. 6*d*. sewed, Bound, 5*s*.]

I Just published, a System of Camp Discipline, Adjutants Duty, Garrison Duty, Regulations for the Land Forces, Kane's Campaigns, and Military History, from 1660 to 1757. with many Copper-plates, 7s 6d.

II. Muller's System of Fortification, Artillery, &c. Cuts, 6 Vol. 1l. 16s.

III Returns Weekly, Monthly, and General, Attestations, &c

IV. New Prussian Field Regulations for Foot, List with Uniforms coloured, and Pay of each Corps in Eng. &c. 19 large fine Plates, 6s. Bound, 7s. 6d.

CONTENTS.

FIELD MARSHALS	Fld M.	General	Lt Gen	M Gen.	Color?
Sir Rob. Rich, Bt	28 Nov 57	29 ... 45	2 July 59	12 ...25	24 Oct. 09
Rd. Vt Molesworth	29 Nov 57	2 Dec 46	do.	19. 9	9 June 19
John Vt. Ligonier	30 Nov 57	3 do	8 1 42-3	2 Jan 39	13 ... 11
COMM. in CHIEF GENERAL.					
C D. of Marlborough			16 July 58	15 Sept 47	30 Mar 45	3 Mar 58

LIEUT. GENERALS	Lt Gen.	Major Gen.	Colorel
Baron de St Hipolite	2 July 1739	12 Nov 1735	
John E. of Westmoreland	do.	16 do.	27 Apl 1715
Sir John Cope	7 Feb. 1742 3	2 Jan 1739	15 Nov. 1711
Roger Handasyd	29 Mar. 1743	co	3 Apr 1712
Henry Hawley	30 do.	do.	16 Oct.
James, Lord Tyrawly	31 do.	do.	29 Jan 1712 13
Charles Otway	28 May 1745	do.	26 July 1717
Charles Lord Cadogan	30 do.	do.	21 Apr. 1719
Philip Arsthuther	31 do.	do.	3 May 1720
James St. Clair	4 June	15 Aug. 1741	26 July 1722
John Guise	7 do.	1 Jan 1741-2	7 July 1724
John Earl of Rothes	5 Aug. 1747	1 Jan 1742-3	29 May 1732
Richard Onslow	6 do.	1 July 1743	10 Jan. 1732-3
Harry Pulteney	8 do.	3 do.	3 Aug. 1733
Hon. Sir Charles Howard	9 do.	4 do.	23 Apr 1734
Philip Bragg	10 do.	5 do.	10 } Oct.
John Huske	11 do.	6 do.	30 }
John Campbell	27 do.	24 Feb 1743-4	}
William Lord Blakeney	11 Sept.	30 Mar. 1745	} 27 June 1737
Humphry Bland	12 do.	do.	}
James Oglethorpe	13 do.	do.	25 } Aug.
John Lord DeLawar	14 do.	do.	20 }
Edward Wolfe	20 do.	27 May	17 Nov. 1739
Hon. Thomas Bligh	23 Mar. 1754	15 Sept. 1747	20 Dec. 1740
Sir John Mordaunt	1 May	22 do.	15 } Jan. 40-1
Hon Ja Cholmondeley	2 do.	23 do.	17 }
John Brown	15 Jan. 1758	26 Mar 1754	1 May 1742
Peregrine Lascelles	16 do.	27 do.	13 } Mar. 42-3
Sir John Bruce Hope, Bt	17 do.	28 do.	15 }
John Folliott	18 do.	30 do	17 } June 1743
Thomas Murray	19 do.	1 Apr.	25 }
Hon. James Stuart	20 do.	1 May	10 July 1744
Lord John Murray	21 do.	16 Feb. 1755	7 } 25 Apr 1745
John Earl of Loudoun	22 do.	17 do.	}
Maurice Bocland	23 do.	18 do.	} 27 May
William E. of Panmure	24 do.	19 do.	}
Lord George Beauclerck	25 do.	20 do	10 do.
Lord George Sackville	26 do.	21 do.	1 }
William Earl of Ancram	27 do.	22 do.	4 } June
Wm. E. of Harrington	28 do.	23 do.	5 }
Hugh Warburton	29 do.	24 do.	22 }

MAJOR GENERALS.	Major Gen.	Colonel	
William Shirley	26 Feb 1755	31 Aug. 1745	} Half Pay
Sir Wm Pepperell, Bt.	27 do.	1 Sept.	
John Duke of Bedford	28 do.	27 do.	
Cuthbert Ellison	1 Mar.	1 Oct.	
Peregrine D. of Ancaster	2 do	4 do.	
Evelyn D of Kingston	3 do.	do.	
John Marq of Granby	4 do.	do.	
Geo E. Cholmondeley	5 do.	do.	R. H. G.
George E of Halifax	6 do.	do.	
Hugh Visc. Falmouth	7 do.	do.	
Simon Earl Harcourt	8 do.	do	
H Arthur E of Powis	9 do	do.	
Rich. Lord Edgecumbe	10 do.	do.	
Michael O'Brien Dilkes	11 do.	14 Nov.	
John Earl of Sandwich	12 do.	22 do.	
W. liam Earl of Home	13 do.	29 do.	
James Kennedy	28 Jan 1756	7 Feb. 1745-6	25 } F. 43 }
Lewis Dejean	29 do.	9 Apr. 1746	3 } H. 4 }
Ho H. Seymour Conway	30 do.	do.	
James Abercromby	31 do.	16 do.	44 F.
Geo. Earl of Albemarle	1 Feb.	24 do.	5 D.
Henry Holmes	2 do.	12 May	31 F.
Sir Edward Agnew Bt.	3 do.	15 Aug.	Gov. of Cliff F.
Robert Napier	4 do.	25 Dec.	12 F.
Sir Rich Lyttelton, Kt. B.	3 Feb. 1757	16 Apr. 1747	
Alexander Dury	4 do.	5 Oct.	1 F. G.
Francis Leighton	5 do.	1 Dec.	32 } F. 36 }
Lord Robert Manners	7 do.	2 do.	
John Mostyn	8 do.	3 do.	13 D.
Edward Pole	9 do.	22 do.	10 F.
Hon. John Waldegrave	10 do.	25 Feb 1747-8	8 D.
Peregrine T. Hopton	11 do.	6 June 1748	40 } F. 24 }
Hon. Edward Cornwallis	12 do.	23 Mar. 1748-9	
Edward Carr	21 do.	27 Apr. 1749	1 F. G.
Lord Charles Hay	22 do.	18 Aug.	33]
Hon. George Boscawen	14 Jan. 1758	18 do.	29 } F. 34]
Tho. Earl of Effingham	15 do.	20 do.	
George Howard	16 do.	21 do.	
Robert Rich	17 do.	22 do.	3 }
Hon. Joseph Yorke	18 do.	1 Nov.	Go. Londonderry
Sir John Whitefoord, Bt.	19 do.	18 Jan. 1749-50	9 F.
William Kingsley	20 do.	11 Apr. 1750	12 D.
Charles Lord Cathcart	21 do.	17 do	20 F.
Paul Mascareen	22 do.	1 June	Brevet
William Whitmore	23 do	29 Jan. 1750-1	53 } F. 4 }
Alexander Duroure	24 do.	27 Feb.	
William Belford	25 do.	8 Mar.	Artillery
Bennet Noel	26 do.	17 Dec. 1751	2 F G.
Granville Elliott	21 Apr.		61 F.

Name	Date	Notes
Toby Keeayrol	15 Feb. 1748	Brevet
Lord George Bentinck	3 Mar. 1752	5 F
John Parfons	4 do	41 F or Inval.
Lord Robert Bertie	do	7 } I. 3 }
John Adlercron	14 do.	
Philip Honywood	17 do.	9 D.
Thomas Dunbar	29 Apr.	Lt Gov of G bialtor
Julius Cæfar	12 May 1753	2 } F G. 1 }
James Durand	22 Dec	
George Wa'fh	22 Jan 1754	45 F
John Campbell	10 Nov. 1755	1+ D.
Daniel Webb	11 do.	1+ } F 2 }
Hon John Fitz-William	12 do	
James Patterfon	19 Dec.	Marines
Andrew Robinfon	24 do	3 F G
Lord Charles Manners	26 do	56 } F. 53 }
Robert Anftruther	28 do.	
William A'Court	29 do.	2 F G.
Charles Montagu	30 do.	59 } F. 76 }
George Lord Forbes	31 do	
John Stanwix	1 Jan 1756	60F Brig in Am 27 Dec 57
Charles Jefferies	3 do.	14 } F. 6 }
James Prevoft	4 do	
William Strode	21 May	6- }
Jeffery Amherft	22 do	Lr of G in Am 1 Mar 58
David Watfon	23 do.	Q. M. G. & Co 65 F
Jofeph Hudfon	24 do.	A de Camp to the King
Hon. John Barrington	25 do.	6- } F 38 }
Sir Ja Lockhart Ror, Bt	26 do.	
Archibald Douglas	27 do.	A de Camp to the King
Robert Armiger	28 do.	65 F
John Griffin Griffin	29 do.	3 F G
Studholm Hodgfon	30 do.	50 F
George Auguftus Elliott	31 do	Aid de Camp to the King
Borgard Michelien	4 Feb. 1757	Artillery
John Forbes	25 do	17 F Brig in Am. 28 Dec 57
Sir David Cunyngha me Bt.	22 Mar.	5- } 51 } F 51 }
John Grey	5 Apl	
Hon. Thomas Brudenell	22 do.	
William Skinner	14 May	Engineer
Edward Whitmore	11 July	22 F } Brig { 30 Dec.57
Charles Lawrence	23 Sept.	60 F } in Am { 31 do
James Wolfe	21 Oct.	6- F } { 20 Jan 58
Robert Monckton	20 Dec	60 F
John Henry B fride	4 Jan. 1758	Engineer
Edward Sandford	23 Mar	52 I.
Theodore Du y	6 Apl.	Marines Brevet
Alexander Ld Lindores	7 do.	81 } F. or Inval. 82 }
John Parker	8 do.	
John Lambton	22 do.	68 } F. 69 }
Hon. Charles Colvill	23 do.	

B 2

COLONELS.

Hon. Sharington Talbot	25 Aug 1758	74 ⎫
John Parflow	27 do.	70 ⎪
William Petitot	29 do.	71 ⎬ F.
William Browre	30 do.	73 ⎪
Hon J Bofcawen	1 May	75 ⎭
John Prideaux	2 do.	3 F G.
George Haldane	3 do.	Brevet
Hon. Thomas Gage	5 do.	80 F Brig in Am. 24 Aug. 58
Hon. George Townfhend	6 do.	Brevet
Ld Frederick Cavendifh	7 do.	⎫ Aid de Camp to the King
Hon. John Weft	8 do.	⎬
Cha Duke of Richmond	9 do	72 F
Henry E of Pembroke	10 do.	
John Severn	7 June	Aid de Camp to the King
John La Fauffille	24 Aug.	Qr M. Gl & Bar.M in Ir, 66 F.

LIEUTENANT-COLONELS.

William Bellenden	3 Apr. 1733	⎫
Charles William Pearce	1 Jan. 1735-6	⎪
Mordaunt Cracherode	15 Dec 1739	⎬ Half P.y
James Cunningham	25 Jan 40-41	⎪
Hugh Macguire	15 Feb	⎭
John Leighton	24 Apr. 1741	Lt Gov Ft Wm.
Nathaniel Mitchell	22 Sept. 1742	Half Pay
Cha Marq of Winchefter	1 May 1745	Lt. of the Tower
John Cofsley	27 do.	Lt. Gov Chelfea Hof.
Boteler Hutchinson	22 June	Half Pay
Arthur Owen	4 Oct	Gov. of Pendennis
Daniel Hering	do.	Half Pay, as Capt. of Foot
Mathew Sewell	do.	Capt. of Invalids
George Vifcount Malpas	do.	Half Pay, as Capt of Foot
John Mordaunt	do.	⎫ Late ⎧ Kingfton's
Gilbert Vane	do.	⎭ ⎩ Berkeley's
Wm Earl of Glencairn	29 Nov	Half Pay
William Dean	17 Feb. 1746	Gov of Upnor Caftle
John Toovey	19 Sept 1747	1 ⎫ D.
John Owen	22 Dec	12 ⎭
John Thomas	17 Feb 1748	2 ⎫ F.G.
Edmund Wynne	22 do.	1 ⎭
Henry Whitley	15 Mar.	10 D.
Juftin Mac Carty	9 Apr.	Half Pay
Chriftopher Clarces	15 Apr. 1749	5 D.
Samuel Bagfhawe	do.	39 F
Thomas Burges	28 do.	3 ⎫ F G
John Seabright	2 May	1 ⎭
George Gray	17 July	1 Tr. H G.
Ja Adolphus Dicken- ⎫ fon Or..ton ⎭	7 Aug.	37 ⎫ F
John Crauford	9 Oct.	13 ⎭
William Ganfell	25 Nov.	2d F. G.
Cyrus Traund	13 Feb 49-50	37 ⎫ F
Sir William Boothby Bt.	19 Mar.	72 ⎭

John

John Gore	11 Apr	1750	3 } 1 } F G.
Hon George Cary	20 Nov.		
Hon James Murray	5 Jan.	1751	15 F. Col. in Am 7 Jan. 1758
John Ferber	29 do		3 } 2 } F G.
Charles Crawe	30 do.		
Thomas Weldon	12 Feb.		41 F. or Invalids
William Lafave	27 do.		24 F
Charles George Clayton	27 Mar.		1 Tr H G G.
Hon William Keppel	28 Apr.		1 F G.
George Wade	31 May		3 D. G.
Hamilton Lambert	28 June		31 F.
Charles Bucknall	2 Sept.		D. Q. M. G & B.
Cecil Forrester	24 Jan.	1752	11 F. (Mr. Irel.
James Forrester	4 Mar.		3 }
John Robinson	15 do.		2 } F. G.
Richard Penson	16 do.		1 }
Marcus Smith	3 June		7 }
Bigoe Armstrong	25 Nov.		18 } F.
John Irwin	27 do.		5 }
William Haviland	16 Dec.		27 F Col. in Am. 9 Jan. 1758
John Clavering	23 do		2 F. G.
Robert Spragge	29 May	1753	49 F.
Hon Chadwal Blayney	8 June		2 }
John Wells	9 do		3 } F. G
Charles Vernon	10 do.		2 }
Marscoe Frederick	11 do.		3 }
R. Dal. Horn Elphinston	20 do.		1 F.
Montagu Blomer	27 Aug.		3 }
Edward Urmston	23 Nov.		1 } F. G.
Wm. Earl of Dalhousie	22 Dec.		1 }
Edward Harvey	5 Jan.	1754	6 D.
Stringer Lawrence	26 Feb.		East Indies
Septimus Robinson	29 May		1 F G.
William Gardner	26 June		11 D
Horatio Sharpe	5 July		West Indies only
William Evelyn	27 Aug.		2d } F. G.
John Salter	28 do		1 }
Thomas Eyle	4 Sept.		14 D.
Richard Worge	4 Oct.		9 F
Ralph Burton	15 do.		48 F. Col. in Am 10 Jan. 1758
James Johnston	2 Dec.		13 D.
James Johnston	17 do.		R Regt II G.
Philip Sherrard	24 Mar.	1755	1 } F G.
Martin Sandys	25 do.		2d }
Robert Clive	31 do		East Indies only
Montagu Wilmot	8 Apr.		40 F. Col. in Am 10 Jan. 1758
Campbell Dalrymple	2 do		
John Littlechales	25 do		
Ruvigny de Cosne	4 Nov.		2d F

George

Name	Date	Regiment
George L... ...arker	5 Nov. 1755	1 F. G.
W...l...m ...ar...on	10 do.	12 }
James G...B...ne	18 do.	10 } F.
Charles ...d...o e	do.	1 H
Nev...l ...r...	do.	1 F. G.
R.chard ...l...l...e	9 Dec.	Marine.
H...n ...s... Stra...	10 do.	4 H.
J...n ...l... ...s	16 do	8 F
...a...t ...c... ...n	17 do.	42 F. Col. in Am 12 Jan 1758
...e...e ...d... ...s	13 do.	26 F.
H...r... ...s... ...	19 do.	2a H.
...a...s ...s...	...0 do.	51 }
...u...n... ...c...ey	?1 do.	52 } F.
...r... ...s...n	2? do.	54 }
W...l...r... ...s...	24 ...o.	1 F Col. in Am. 12 Jan. 1758
Pet... ...e...	26 do.	56 }
Ch... s ...c...	27 do.	46 }
Th...s ...k.nson	28 do.	36 } F.
B...am C... ...s	29 do.	4 }
William Augustus Pitt	30 do.	59 }
John Scott	31 do.	3 }
George Bodens	1 Jan. 1756	2 } F. G.
Lord Adam Gordon	2 do	3 }
Henry Bouquet	3 do.	2 }
Frederick Haldiman	4 do.	60 F. Col. { 16 Jan. 58
Sir John St. Clair, Bt.	6 do.	in Am. { 17 do.
John Reed	7 do.	{ 18 do.
Robert Scott	8 do.	34 }
Edward Sacheverell Pole	9 do.	6 } F.
Owen Wynne	9 do.	23 }
William Deny	18 May	9 D.
James Muir Campbell	2 June	America only
Robert Campbell	3 do.	2 Dr. G.
William Alexand. Sorell	4 do.	3 }
Richard Lambert	5 do.	2 } F.G.
Alexander Maitland	6 do.	1 }
Henry Richardson	23 do.	1 }
Arthur Morris	21 Sept.	29 F
Andrew Lord Rollo	22 Nov.	17 F. } Co in Am { 19 Jan 58
James Molesworth	do.	22 F. } { 20 do
John Pomeroy	do.	2 }
Hon Arch. Montgomery	4 Jan. 1757	61 } F.
Simon Frafer	5 do.	77 } F. Co in Am. { 21 Jan 58
Benjamin Carpenter	18 do.	78 } { 22 do.
Demetrius James	2 Feb.	2 Tr. H. G
Hunt Walsh	do.	4? } F. Co. in Am. } 23 Jan 58
John Laborde	do.	28 } } 24 do.
George Williamson	3 do.	16 F.
Thomas Desaguliers	4 do.	} Artil. Col. in Am 25 Jan. 58
George Preston	25 do.	2 Dr.

George

Name	Date	Regiment/Note
George Scott	22 Mar. 1757	25 } F
Thomas Lil'er	5 Apr.	14 }
John Young	26 do	60 F Col in Am. 26 Jan. 1758
William Cuninghame	7 May	3 F. G.
George Lawson Hall	14 do	7 Dr.
Guy Carleton	18 June	72 F
Charles Hotham	25 do	Deputy Adjutant General
William Thomson	13 July	1 D. G
Francis Desmarette	15 do.	2 T H G.
William Napier	27 do.	3 Horse
Thomas Townshend	3 Aug.	57 F.
Robert Clerk	8 do.	Brevet
William Diaper	2 Nov.	79 F.
Robert Cuninghame	3 do	Brevet
Hon. William Howe	17 Dec	58 F. Col. in Am. 27 Jan 1758
John Bradstreet	27 do.	Dep Qr Mr. Gl. in Am.
James Montresor	4 Jan. 1758	Engineer
William Arnot	31 do.	53 F.
Hon. Robert Brudenell	do	3 F G.
Hon. Roger Townshend	1 Feb.	D. Adj. Gl. and Col in Am.
Henry Fletcher	16 do	35 } (24 Aug 58
John Handfield	18 Mar.	40 } F.
John Hale	19 do.	47 }
Robert Boyd	25 do.	Brevet
Macpherson Neale	7 Apr.	3 } F.G.
Geo Marq. of Blandford	8 do.	1 }
Robert Douglas	10 do	19 ⌉
Wollaston Pym	11 do.	64	
William Tayler	12 do.	71	
Charles Vignoles	13 do	70	
Nehemiah Donnellan	14 do.	58	
John Jennings	15 do.	62	F.
John Salt	16 do.	65	
Peter Desbrisay	17 do.	63	
John Barlow	18 do.	61	
William Wilkinson	19 do.	50	
Jorden Wren	20 do.	75	
John Beckwith	21 do.	20 ⌋
James Burleigh	22 do.	Marines
William Adey	do.	68 ⌉
Rowland Phillips	23 do	66	
John Browne	24 do.	69	
William Masters	25 do.	74	F.
Robert Robinson	26 do.	67	
Hezekiah Fleming	27 do.	73	
Edward Maxwell	do.	21 ⌋
Francis Craig	28 do.	2 ⌉
William Williams	29 do	3	
Bernard Hale	30 do	3	F. G.
Lancelot Baugh	1 May	1	
Rowland Alston	2 do	1 ⌋

William

William Style	3 May 1758	1 ⎫
Henry Lifter	4 do.	2 ⎬ F. G.
Henry Clinton	6 do.	1 ⎭
Robert Watfon	7 do.	Dep. Quarter-Mafter Gen.
Ld. Geo. Henry Lennox	8 do	33 F.
Charles Fitz Roy	9 do.	1 ⎫ F. G.
John Burgoyne	10 do.	2 ⎭
William M'Dowall	26 June	32 F.
James Robertfon	8 July	Dep Qr.-Mr.General in Am.
Arthur Graham	24 Aug.	1 F. G.

M A J O R S.

Richard Bowles	13 Mar. 1741-2	81 F.
Sir Charleton Leighton Bt	1 May 1745	Half Pay
Charles H. Collins	4 Oct.	Major to T. of Lond.
William Johnfton	do.	82 F.
William Hepburn	do.	Captain 2 D.
Thomas Bate	do.	⎫ On Half Pay
Robert Mitford	do.	⎭
Chiverton Hartop	do.	Captain 41 F.
George Marriott	do.	Captain 6 D.
Mathew Swiney	do.	Montague s
Scot Floyer	do.	Late Gower's
Charles Durand	29 Nov	On Half Pay
William Brown	12 May 1746	81 F.
James Otway	26 Feb 1747-8	⎫ On Half Pay
Charles Duterme	26 Aug.	⎭
Edward Strode	12 Feb. 1750-1	41 F
Henry Hart	3 Mar.	Lieut Gr. Sheernefs
William Godfrey	4 do	82 F
William Fitz-Thomas	31 May	3 ⎫ D. G.
William Eaft	11 Oct. 1752	2 ⎭
Samuel Brown	12 do.	4 D
Park Pepper	29 May 1753	49 F.
Digby Berkeley	11 June	Captain of Invalids
William Hill	12 Mar. 1754	5 D
William Farquhar	do	15 F.
Nathaniel Bateman	5 June	⎫ 1 Tr. H. G.
Philip Jennings	21 Aug.	⎭
John Balaguire	4 Sept.	13 Dr.
Charles Craven	24 Co.	Half Pay
Bartholomew Gallatin	1 Dec.	1 D
John Chalmers	1 Mar 1755	Artillery
R. Rickart Hepbourn	25 Apr.	6 D.
Flower Mocher	5 July	2 Tr H G G.
Alexander Murray	1 Oct.	45 F
James Kinneer	25 do.	Half Pay, late 50 F.
Francis Forde	13 Nov.	39 F.
John Wynne	18 do.	12 D
Hector Boifrand	9 Dec.	⎫ Marines
John Mackenzie	10 do.	⎭
Henry Holmes	do.	4 H.

Bartholomew

Name	Date	Regiment
Bartholomew Blake	10 Dec. 1755	29 } Foot
Eyre Maffey	do.	27 }
Philip Roberts	do.	1 H.
John Purcell Kempe	11 do.	Marines
John Bell	13 do.	14 }
Sir R. Hamilton, Bart.	14 do.	18 } Foot
Noel Furye	16 do.	51 }
Hugh Morgan	18 do.	52 }
Samuel Boucher	20 do.	Marines
David Erfkine	22 do.	26 } Foot
John Doyne	27 do.	56 }
Robert Sloper	28 do.	10 D.
Henry Gore	30 do.	7 F.
Marcus Norman	2 Jan. 1756	14 D.
Joseph Lewis Feyrac	5 do.	59 }
William Eyres	7 do.	44 }
Robert Melvill	8 do.	38 } Foot.
Auguftine Prevoft	9 do.	60 }
Sir Hu. Williams, Bart.	10 do.	6 }
Thomas Hardy	11 do.	4 }
Charles Bradfhaigh	23 Mar.	1 Tr. H. G. G.
Edward Clayton	9 Apr.	9 }
Francis Bonham	5 May	3 } Dr.
George Warde	2 June	11 }
Edward Rycaut	10 do.	Marines
William Pieft on	26 Aug.	24 }
James Vignoles	28 do.	31 }
Cholmeley Scot	30 do.	11 }
Peter Daulhat	1 Sept.	33 }
Shuckburgh Hewett	3 do.	3 }
John Cook	4 do.	8 } Foot
Corbet Parry	6 do.	12 }
Thomas Marlay	7 do.	23 }
Joseph Higginfon	8 do.	62 }
John Darby	21 do.	17 }
William Lufhington	22 Nov.	8 Dr.
William Newton	do.	76 F.
William Blackett	do.	Capt. of Invalds
Peter Chefter	do.	76 } Foot
Edward Windus	do.	2 }
Hugh Forbes	17 Dec.	R. Regt. H. G.
Richard Prefcott	20 do.	72 }
James Clephane	4 Jan. 1757	78 }
James Grant	5 do.	77 } Foot
John Campbell	6 do.	78 }
Alexander Campbell	7 do.	77 }
Gervas Remington	18 do.	36 }
Lewis Ch. Montolieu	do.	2 Tr. H G
John Dundas	2 Feb.	34 } Foot
Joseph Gabbett	do.	16 }

John

John Dalling	2 Feb 1757	28 } Foot
Robert Elliott	do.	4 ;
William Browning	do.	46
Thomas Flight	4 do.	Artillery
Hamilton Blair	9 Mar.	2 Dr.
Thomas Goodricke	22 do.	25 }
David Chapeau	5 Apr.	13 } Foot
John Tullikens	26 do.	60
Frederick Hamilton	7 May	1
John Richardson	13 July	1 Dr. G.
Robert Sloughter	15 do.	2 Tr. H. G.
George Onslow	3 Aug.	57 F.
John Rutter	27 do.	3 H.
Cholmondeley Brereton	2 Nov.	79 }
William Eustace	17 do.	5 } Foot
Hon. George Monson	18 do.	79
John Lind	28 do.	Capt. of Invalids
James Agnew	17 Dec.	58 Foot
Archibald Patoun	4 Jan. 1758	} Engineer
Patrick Mackellar	do.	
Hans Musgrave	12 do.	9 } Foot
John Lindsay	31 do.	53
John Litchfield	10 Feb.	7 Dr.
Arthur Preston	11 do.	2 H.
Roger Morris	16 do.	35 Foot
John Tufton Mason	20 do.	Marines
Christopher Aldridge	18 Mar.	40
John Hussey	19 do.	47
Robert Ross	20 do.	43
Edward Martin	22 Apr.	69
Charles Lumisden	23 do.	19
Robert Murray	24 do.	71
Thomas Ball	25 do.	64
Thomas Shirley	26 do.	73
James Stuart	27 do.	75
James Ramsay	28 do.	30
John Del Garno	29 do.	65
John Trollope	30 do.	63
Robert Hall	1 May	37 } Foot
Lewis Thomas	2 do.	50
Christopher Teesdale	3 do.	61
Thomas Maule	4 do.	74
Robert Pigot	5 do.	70
William Napier	6 do.	68
Charles Beauclerck	7 do.	66
Adam Levingston	8 do.	21
John Maxwell	do.	20
Alexander M'Dowall	9 do.	67
Robert Walsh	10 do.	54
David Lindsay	27 do.	1
James Seton	26 June	32
Robert Wrey		22
Daniel Chenevix	24 Aug.	Irish Artillery

Rank.	Name	Rank in the	
		Troop	Army
Capt. & Colonel	John Lord De Lawarr	30 Aug 1737	L. Gen. 14 Sep 47
1ſt Lt. & Lt. Col.	George Grav	17 July 1719	
2d Lt. & Lt. Col.	Hon John Weſt	8 Aug. 1755	Col 8 May 1 8
Cornet & Major	Nathaniel Bateman	21 Aug. 1754	5 June 1754
Guidon & Major	Philip Jennings	do.	
Exempt & Capt.	{ Thomas Twyſden	9 Apr 1748	
	Edward Sneyd	5 June 1754	
	James Dunne	21 Aug.	
	William Culling	5 June 1758	
Brigadier & Lieut.	{ Peter Sheppard	9 Apr 1748	
	James Rolt	12 June 1749	
	John Shore	5 June 1754	
	James D'Auvergne	5 June 1758	
Adjutant & Lieut.	Peter Hawker	5 June 1758	
Sub-Brigadier and Cornet	{ John Croft	5 June 1754	
	Charles Lanoe	17 Dec.	
	Tho Dufour Eaton	13 Nov. 1756	
	James Mawhood	5 June 1758	

Chaplain . . . William Greaves 25 Jan. 1741-2
Surgeon . . . Ab. Wh. Humphreys 21 June 1756

Agent, Mr. Richardſon, Downing-Street, Weſtminſter.

N. B. *The Officers who have no Dates in the Column of Rank in the Army, take Rank by their Commiſſions, in the Troop or Regiment.*

C

Second

Rank.	Name.	Rank in the	
		Troop.	*Army.*
Capt & Colonel	Cha. Lord Cadogan	25 April 1743	L. Gen. 30 May 45
1ſt Lt & Lt. Col.	Benjamin Carpenter	15 July 1757	18 Jan. 1757
2d Lt. & Lt. Col.	Francis Deſmarette	15 do.	
Cornet & Major	Lew. Ch. Montolieu	15 July 1757	18 Jan. 1757
Guidon & Major	Robert Sloughter	15 do.	
Exempt & Capt.	Felix Buckley	22 July 1751	
	G. Fr. Cunningham	2 Dec. 1754	
	Richard Bowles	18 Jan. 1757	
	Oliver Stephens	15 July	
Brigadier & Lieut.	Charles Clarke	2 Dec. 1754	27 Aug. 1754
	Edward Maurice	14 Oct. 1755	2 Dec.
	Samuel Pocock	18 Jan. 1757	
	Robert Hinde	15 July	
Adjutant & Lieut.	John Wheatland	14 Oct. 1755	
Sub-Brigadier and Cornet	William Egerton	11 Jan. 1755	
	Rupert Clarke	18 Jan 1757	
	Claud Benezet	9 Mar.	
	W. J. Spencer Waſey	15 July	7 Oct. 1756
Chaplain . .	Thomas Rayne	20 Dec. 1740	
Surgeon . .	Duncan Forbes	14 June 1756	

Agent, Mr. Winter, Brewer-Street.

First

Rank.	Name	Rank in the	
		Troop.	Army
Capt. & Col.	Ho. Richard Onflow	25 April 1745	L. Gen. 6 Aug. 47
Lt & Lt Col.	Courthorpe Clayton	23 Mar 1756	27 Mar. 1751
Major	Charles Bradfhaigh	23 Mar. 1756	
Lt. & Capt.	{ John Jeffreys { Edward Fletcher	13 Sept. 1754 25 Mar. 1756	25 Apr. 1751 13 Sept. 1754
Guidon & Capt.	Jofeph Walford	23 Mar. 1756	
Sub-Lieut.	{ Wm. Harris Jeffreys { John Hare	9 Dec 1755 23 Mar 1756	26 Sept. 1754 5 Mar. 1755
Adj. & Sub-Lt.	John Bateman	18 May 1756	
Chaplain	James Sanvey	26 Jan. 1747-8	
Surgeon	John Ruding	9 Nov. 1747	

Agent, Mr. Calcraft, Channel-Row.

| Rank. | Name. | Rank in the | |
		Troop.	Army.
Capt & Col.	Wm. E. of Harrington	5 June 1745	Lt. Gen. 28 Jan. 58
Lt & Lt Col.	Geo. Auguf Elliot	18 May 1747	Col 31 May 1756
Major	Flower Mocher	5 July 1754	
Lt & Capt	{ Paul Pechell { James Harrington	5 July 1755 1 Oct.	12 Dec. 1746 5 July 1755
Guidon & Capt.	James Bellenden	1 Oct. 1755	8 Mar. 1747-8
Sub-Lieut.	{ George Ainflie { Charles Smythe	8 Aug. 1755 25 Dec.	24 Dec. 1755
Adj. & Sub-Lt.	Philip Ainflie	23 Mar. 1754	
Chaplain	Edward Fleet	26 Dec. 1750	
Surgeon	Jofeph Elfe	11 Feb. 1756	

Agent, Mr. Fifher, Axe-Yard, Weftminfter.

Royal

Rank.	Name.	Rank in the	
		Regiment	Army.
Colonel	John Marq of Granby	13 May 1758	M Gen. 4 Mar 1755
Lieut. Col	James Johnson	17 Dec 1754	
Major	Hugh Forbes	17 Dec. 1756	
Captain -	John Keilet	17 Dec 1754	
	Frecheville Ramsden	26 Feb. 1755	
	Henry Stubbs	23 Aug.	
	Andrew Forbes	17 Dec. 1756	
	Wynter Blathwayt	5 Apr. 1757	
	Edward Ligonier	10 Feb 1758	29 July 1757
Capt Lieut	Alex Ld Rutherford	5 Apr. 1757	
Lieutenant -	Pairavacini Mawhood	29 Oct. 1754	
	George Bowles	20 Feb 1755	
	Charles Tufnall	23 Aug.	
	Pat Warrender	14 June 1756	
	Richard Onslow	8 Dec.	
	Walter Thrufby	17 do.	
	Tho. Chamberlaine	28 Sept. 1757	
	Urban Hall	8 May 1758	
Cornet - -	Frederick Evelyn	14 June 1756	
	William Middleton	7 Dec	
	Alexander Campbell	8 do	
	Edward Lascelles	17 do	
	William Mailares	27 Dec. 1757	
	Jonn Walfh	26 Jan. 1758	
	Daniel Davenport	8 May	
	Joseph Bedford	9 do	
	Richard Bulstrode	19 June	
Chaplain	Richard Levett	5 Apr 1748	
Adjutant	Henry Stubbs	22 Mar 1743	
Surgeon	William Mitchell	24 Apr. 1750	

Agent, Mr Calcraft, Channel-Row, Westminster.

First

| Rank. | Name. | Rank in the | |
		Regiment.	Army
Colonel -	John Brown	1 Apr. 1743	L. Gen. 15 Jan. 1758
Lieut Col.	Charles *Lord* Moore	18 Nov. 1755	
Major -	Philip Roberts	10 Dec. 1755	
Captain -	{ Joſeph White { Chriſtopher Parker { John Aſhburnham	26 May 1747 15 Mar. 1755 10 Dec.	
Capt Lieut.	Robert Wallis	10 Dec. 1755	
Lieutenant -	{ Thomas Kenrick { Hon Hu Skeffington { John Ellwood { Rich. Rochfort { Wilkinſon Smith	11 May 1748 12 Mar. 1754 9 Apr. 1756 27 July 27 May 1758	
Cornet -	{ Holland Leckie { John Croker { Clotworthy Rowley { Richard Warren { Jeffrey Brown { Lord Delvin	10 Dec. 1755 do. 9 Apr 1756 8 Mar. 1757 27 July 27 May 1758	
Chaplain -	Peter Weſterra	4 Sept. 1754	
Adjutant -	Alexander Cox	15 Mar. 1755	
Surgeon -	Robert Leſter	16 Feb. 1756	

Agent, Mr Deſbriſay, Dublin

Second

		Rank in the	
Rank.	*Name.*	*Regiment.*	*Army.*
Colonel -	Hon. Thomas Bligh 22 Dec. 1747		Lt. Gen. 23 Mar. 54
Lieut. Col.	Henry Stamer	19 Dec 1755	
Major -	Arthur Preston	11 Feb. 1758	
Captian	{ Robert Sandford Henry Wallis Thomas Pope	16 Feb. 1756 27 Apr. 11 Feb. 1758	
Capt. Lieut.	Edward Conyers	27 Apr. 1756	
Lieutenant	{ Arthur Fitzgerald James Moore Guy Moore Nicholas Fitzgerald Patrick Webb	14 Ju'y 1749 12 Mar. 1754 15 Mar. 1755 10 Dec 11 Feb. 1758	
Cornet	{ John Jenkinson John Nugent Bryan Mansergh William Buttle Char. Lennox Smith William Stearn Noy	27 Nov 1752 12 May 1754 10 Dec 1755 27 Apr 1756 11 Feb 1758 27 May	
Chaplain Adjutant Surgeon	Arthur Champagne Thomas Pope Francis Whetstone	10 Dec 1755 3 June 1757 Feb. 1721	

Agent, Mr. Desbrisay, Dublin.

Third

Rank.	Name	Rank in the Regiment.	Army.
Colonel -	Lewis Dejean	5 Apr 1757	M. Gen. 29 Jan. 56
Lieut. Col. -	William Naper	27 July 1757	
Major -	John Rutter	27 Aug 1757	
Captain -	John Skottowe Wm Phineas Bowles Edward Afhenhurft	8 Apr. 1755 14 July 1756 8 Mar. 1757	
Capt. Lieut.	St. Geo. Richardfon	14 July 1756	
Lieutenant -	John Reynell Thomas Defbrifay Samuel Ball Thomas Brown Gilbert Mellifont	4 Sept. 1754 8 Apr. 1755 10 Dec. 8 Mar. 1757 12 Jan. 1758	
Cornet - -	Benjamin Bunbury Richard Bowater Francis Caulfield John Lovet Philip Tuite Ifaac Maddock	4 Sept. 1754 8 Apr. 1755 10 Dec 8 Mar. 1757 12 Jan 1758 31 Mar.	
Chaplain -	A. V. De, Voeux	2 Nov. 1742	
Adjutant -	Henry Peterkin	3 June 1752	
Surgeon -	Robert Breviter	16 Dec. 1753	

Agent, Mr.   Dublin.

Rank.	Name.	Rank in the	
		Regiment	Army.
Colonel -	Ho. H. Seym. Conway	8 July 1754	M Gen 30 Jan. 56
Lieut. Col.	Hon. Francis Stuart	10 Dec. 1755	
Major -	Henry Holmes	10 Dec. 1755	
Captain -	Hon. Henry Stuart	26 Mar. 1747	
	Arthur Graham	16 Oct. 1748	
	Wm. Cuninghame	11 Feb. 1758	
Captain Lieut.	Henry Gore	11 Feb. 1758	
Lieutenant	William Lovett	10 Dec. 1755	
	Thomas Webber	10 Feb. 1758	
	Anthony Cliffe	11 do.	
	Edward Loftus	26 May	
	Robert Doyne	27 do.	
Cornet -	Charles Boyle	10 Dec. 1755	
	William Roberts	28 May 1756	
	Michael Head	10 Feb. 1758	
	John Staples	11 do	
	Thomas Pigott	26 May	
	Nicholas Loftus	27 do.	
Chaplain	George Prefton	20 Aug 1751	
Adjutant	Thomas Webber	3 June 1752	
Surgeon	Stephen Moore	25 Feb. 1741	

Agent, Mr Chaigneau. Dublin

Rank.	Name.	Rank in the	
		Regiment.	Army
Colonel - -	Humphry Bland	8 July 1752	Lt Gen. 12 Sept. 47
Lieut Col. -	Wm. Thomson	13 July 1757	
Major - -	John Richardson	13 July 1757	
Captain - -	Sandys Mill	8 Mar. 1747-8	
	Charles Hamilton	12 Mar 1755	
	William Lightfoot	25 Dec.	
	Thicke Brace	20 Dec 1756	
	Richard Callis	12 Jan. 1757	
	Martin Tucker	13 July	
	John Fletcher	7 Apr. 1758	
Captain Lieut.	John Floyd	12 Jan. 1757	
Lieutenant -	Richard Wolseley	22 July 1751	
	Leonard Jacob	19 June 1752	
	George Lewis	12 Oct.	
	Richard Porter	25 Dec. 1755	
	Clifton Rading	26 do.	
	Robert Hodgson	20 Dec. 1756	
	John Threlfall	12 Jan. 1757	
	Charles Morris	13 July	
	Nevil Bland	7 Apr. 1758	
Cornet - -	Henry Howard	30 Mar. 1755	
	Robert Lukin	25 Dec.	
	Richard Downes	26 do.	
	Hoie Browse Truste	27 do.	
	William Hope Weir	5 Sept 1756	
	John Prince	20 Dec.	
	Fra. Laprimaudaye	27 Jan. 1757	
	Benjamin Lewis	13 July	
	Sir J. St Clair, Bart.	20 Dec.	
	Andrew Wauchope	22 July 1758	
Chaplain	W. Dob Humphreys	10 Feb. 1753	
Adjutant	John Prince	do.	
Surgeon	Thomas Mills	18 Feb 1723	

Agent, Mr. Lamb, Brook-treet.

Rank.	Name.	Rank in the	
		Regim.	Army
Colonel - -	Ld. Geo. Sackville	5 April 1755	L. Gen 26 Jan. 1758
Lieut. Col. -	Jam. Muir Campbell	7 May 1757	2 June 1756
Major - -	William East	11 Oct. 1752	
Captain - -	Hon. Ja. Somerville	26 Jan. 1750-1	
	William Arnot	12 Oct. 1752	
	Hon. Hu. Somerville	29 May 1753	
	John Ferguson	25 Dec. 1755	
Captain Lieut.	William Innes	25 Dec. 1755	
Lieutenant -	Edmund Cox	25 Jan. 1750-1	
	Thomas Mallack	12 Oct. 1752	
	Joseph Smallman	27 Nov.	
	Francis Cooke	25 Dec. 1755	
	William Beckwith	26 do.	
	Francis Travell	6 Aug. 1757	
Cornet - -	John Kirkpatrick	29 May 1753	25 Feb. 1755-6
	Henry Legard	26 Dec. 1755	
	Edward Brudenell	18 Jan. 1757	
	William Smith	6 August	
	James Cathcart	8 May 1758	
	John Caulfield	9 do	
	Richard Hinde	10 do.	
Chaplain - -	Richard Davies	14 Ap. 1756	
Adjutant - -	Joseph Smallman	6 Feb. 1756-7	
Surgeon - -	Francis Tomkins	3 Sept. 1751	

Rank	Name.	Rank in the	
		Regiment.	Army.
Colonel - -	Sir Charles Howard	15 Mar. 47-8	Lt. Gen. 9 Aug. 47
Lieut. Col. -	George Wade	31 May 1751	
Major - -	Will. Fitz-Thomas	31 May 1751	
Captain - -	Edward Milbanke	16 Apr. 1747	4 Oct. 1745
	Charles Chauncy	25 Nov. 1754	31 July 1749
	Thomas Reynolds	12 Nov. 1755	
	William Lawley	25 Dec.	
Captain Lieut.	Æneas M'Donald	23 Mar. 1756	
Lieutenant -	John Manfell	25 Dec. 1755	1 Jan. 1756
	Robert Brittan	26 do.	
	Robert Waller	22 Mar. 1756	
	Edward Ball	3 Sept.	
	Wade Caulfield	12 Oct.	
	Henry Sanger	28 Nov. 1757	
Cornet - -	John Wogan	25 Feb. 1756	
	Hen. Will Guion	26 do.	
	Henry Knight	4 Mar.	
	Ralph Abercrombie	23 do.	
	Thomas Allen	3 Sept.	
	Philip De la Motte	26 Oct	
	Richard Grant	28 Nov. 1757	
Chaplain - -	Thomas Hefkett		
Adjutant -	Henry Sanger	29 Oct. 1753	
Surgeon - -	Abraham Godfrey	28 Mar. 1751	

Agent, Mr. Adair, Pall-Mall.

First

Rank.	Name.	Rank in the	
		Regiment	Army.
Colonel - -	Henry Hawley	10 May 1740	L. Gen. 30 Mar. 43
Lieut. Col. -	John Toovey	2 Dec. 1754	19 Sept 1747
Major - -	Bartholom. Gallatin	1 Dec 1754	
Captain - -	Richard Burton	30 Oct. 1751	
	Robert Winde	31 do	
	Sampson Barber	2 Dec. 1754	
	George Warrender	25 Dec. 1755	
Captain Lieut.	John Davies	25 Dec. 1755	
Lieutenant -	Wiltshire Wilson	3 Mu 49 50	
	James Defmarette	28 June 1751	
	Edward Coleman	2 Dec 1754	
	Charles Mawhood	8 Nov. 1756	
	Henry De Vic	17 Dec.	
	John Fremantle	11 Jan. 1758	2 Oct 1755
Cornet - -	William Wolfley	25 Mar 1755	
	John Ballantyne	25 Dec.	2 Apr 1746
	James Langham	8 Nov. 1756	
	Philip Goldfworthy	17 Dec.	
	Sir W Manfell Bart.	28 Jan 1757	
	Randolph Knipe	7 May	
	—— Duffe	20 Dec.	
Chaplain - -	George Tilfon	23 July 1748	
Adjutant - -	Sampfon Barber	15 June 1743	
Surgeon - -	Ch. Wilfon Lyon	10 Nov. 1750	

Agent, Mr. Rofs, Conduit-Street.

Rank	Name.	Rank in the	
		Regiment.	Army.
Colonel - -	John Campbell	29 Apr. 1752	L Gen. 27 Aug. 47
Lieut. Col. -	George Preston	25 Feb. 1757	
Major - -	Hamilton Blair	9 Mar 1757	
Captain - -	William Hepburne	24 July 1754	Major 4 Oct. 1745
	John Douglas	11 Jan. 1755	
	Francis Lindsay	25 Dec.	
	Hon. Will. Napier	9 Mar. 1757	
Captain Lieut.	William Bury	9 Mar. 1757	
Lieutenant -	Mungo Law	13 Sept. 1754	
	Alex. Conyngham	26 Feb. 1755	
	Henry Moore	25 Dec.	
	Edward Blackett	26 do.	
	David Home	9 Mar. 1757	
	Basil Heron	8 July 1758	
Cornet - -	John Mitchell	18 Nov. 1755	
	John Forbes	25 Dec.	
	James Colhoun	26 July 1756	
	John Campbell	12 Jan. 1757	31 Aug. 1756
	Thomas Fowke	9 Mar.	
	Charles Scott	8 May 1758	
Chaplain - -	Walter Paterson	8 July 1752	
Adjutant - -	John Forbes	31 May 1755	
Surgeon - -	Wm Mc. Kerrall	26 Oct 1756	

Agent, Mr. Calcraft, Channel-Row, Westminster.

Third

Rank.	Name	Rank in the	
		Regiment	Army.
Colonel, - -	G. E. of Albemarle	8 Apr. 1755	M. Gen. 1 Feb. 56
Lieut. Col. -	Campb. Dalrymple	24 Apr. 1755	
Major - -	Francis Bonham	5 May 1756	
Captain - -	Charles Byne Wm de St. Amour Ant St. Leger Jenkins Reading	24 Dec 1755 25 do. 5 May 1756 7 Oct.	
Captain Lieut.	James Irvine	5 May 1756	
Lieutenant -	Henry Stanley Richard Ward Tho. Alex Fuller Godfr Woodw Vane John Melles Silvester Richmond	10 Feb. 1753 25 Dec. 1755 23 Mar. 1756 5 May 9 July 7 Oct.	3 Oct. 1755
Cornet - -	John Tonyn John Clegg Jocelyn Price George Moreland James Barker Basil Beridge Francis Moreland	25 Dec. 1755 26 do. 5 May 1756 12 do. 9 July 8 July 1757 25 Mar 1758	8 Aug. 1755 27 Dec. 1755
Chaplain - -	Thomas Beighton	6 Aug 1742	
Adjutant - -	John Clegg	18 Feb 1746-7	
Surgeon - -	William Hocke	8 July 1752	

Agent, M. Adair, Pall mall.

Fourth

| Rank. | Name. | Rank in the | |
		Regiment.	Army.
Colonel - -	Sir Robert Rich Bt.	13 May 1735	F. Mar. 28 Nov. 57
Lieut. Col. -	Archibald Douglas	4 Feb. 1746-7	Col. 27 May 1756
Major - -	Samuel Brown	12 Oct. 1752	
Captain - -	John Bradford	5 Mar 1750-1	
	James Tindal	12 Oct. 1752	
	Edward Griffith	25 Dec. 1755	
	Thomas Adams	8 May 1758	
Captain Lieut.	James Hugonin	26 Jan. 1758	
Lieutenant -	John Hamilton	9 Dec 1755	
	David Barclay	26 do.	
	Richard Ellis	25 Feb. 1757	
	George Armytage	26 do.	
	Ralph Dundas	26 Jan. 1758	
	Francis Jefferson	8 May	
Cornet - -	Duke Adams	9 Dec. 1755	
	James Boyd	25 do.	
	Francis Jenison	26 do.	
	Emanuel Walton	5 Apr. 1757	
	Herbert Price	22 do.	
	Thomas Hewan	7 Mar. 1758	
	Joseph Turnpenny	8 May	
Chaplain - -	William Smythies	12 Feb 1750-1	
Adjutant - -	James Boyd	2 July 1747	
Surgeon - -	James Baddeley	20 May 1752	

Agent, Mr. Guerin, Crown Court, Westminster.

Rank.	Name.	Regiment.	Rank in the Army.
Colonel	Rd. Vif. Molefworth	27 June 1757	F Mar. 29 Nov 57
Lieut. Col.	Chriftopher Clarges	20 Feb. 1749-50	15 Apr. 1749
Major	William Hill	12 Mar. 1754	
Captain	Hugh Cane	12 Mar. 1754	28 Oct. 1745
	Cuthbert Smith	do.	
	Richard Gorges	27 Apr. 1756	
	George Clarges	22 June 1757	
	William Rofs	15 Oct.	
	Wm Ld. Newbattle	21 Nov.	
Captain Lieut.	St. Geo. Stevenfon	15 Oct. 1757	
Lieutenant	Phil. Ormfby	15 Apr 1749	1 May 1743
	Hen. Mark Mafon	4 Jan. 1749-50	
	Robert Molefworth	27 Nov. 1752	
	William Shean	16 Dec.	
	Edward Young	16 Feb. 1756	
	John Nicholls	28 May	
	John Creighton	8 Mar 1757	
	Richard Wolfe	15 Oct	
Cornet	Nathaniel Mitchell	10 Mar 1753	11 Dec. 1752
	Henry Jenny	12 Mar. 1754	
	Harry Percy Monk	22 Jan 1755	
	Thomas Vetey	16 Feb. 1756	
	Gilbert Toler	do.	
	Bartholom Purdon	28 May	
	Benjamin Lucas	8 Mar. 1757	
	John Butlock	15 Oct.	
	William Caulfield	17 Dec.	
Chaplain	Ralph Cocking	21 Oct 1729	
Adjutant	Richard Wolfe		
Surgeon	Alex Crommelin	28 Aug. 1753	

Agent, M. Dobson, Dublin

Rank	Name.	Rank in the	
Reg.l	Name.	Regiment.	Army.
Colonel - -	Ho Ja Cholmondeley	16 Jan. 49-50	Lt. Gen. 2 May 54
Lieut Col.	Edward Harvey	29 May 1754	5 Jan. 1754
Major - -	Rt. Richard Hepburn	25 Apr. 1755	
Captain - -	Patrick Tonyn George Marriott James Suttle John Whitmore	10 May 1751 29 May 1754 24 Apr. 1755 25 Dec.	Major 4 Oct. 1745
Captain Lieut.	John Robins	25 Dec 1755	
Lieutenant -	Drury Jones Richard Edwards Edward Arblaster William Hartnell John Elliot Guft. Guydickens	19 Feb 1754 24 Apr. 1755 1 Oct. 14 do. 26 Dec. 2 Sept. 1756	1 Sept. 1745
Cornet - -	Edward Walpole Edward Lovell Hon. John Sandys John Whitefoord John Webster Clement Newsham Henry Sayer	14 Oct 1755 9 Dec. 25 do. 2 Sept. 1756 4 Jan. 1757 5 do. 5 Apr.	25 July 1748
Chaplain - -	Charles Burdett	26 Nov. 1751	
Adjutant - -	John Webster	14 Apr. 1756	
Surgeon - -	Charles Launder	9 Mar 1746-7	

Agent, Mr. Walmesley, Scotland-Yard.

Seventh

			Rank in the	
Rank.	*Name.*	*Regt.*	*Army.*	
Colonel - -	Sir John Cope	12 Aug. 1741	Lt Gen 7 Feb. 42-3
Lieut. Col. -	Geo. Lawfon Hall	14 May 1757	
Major - -	John Litchfield	10 Feb. 1758	
Captain - -	William Erfkine	25 Dec 1755	11 June 1756
	Thomas Hay	14 May 1757	
	John Brown	10 Feb. 1758	
	Ruffel Manners	do	
Captain Lieut.	William Ball	25 Dec. 1755	
Lieutenant -	William Thornton	4 Mar. 1752	
	Rowland Johnfon	10 Feb 1753	
	Pelham Maitland	29 May	
	Lewis Francis Irwin	30 Mar. 1754	
	Jonath. Scott	28 June 1756	
	John Ballmer	14 May 1757	
Cornet - -	Samuel Bayley	29 May 1753	
	Thomas Bland	30 Mar. 1754	
	Alexander Hay	25 Dec. 1755	
	John Jennings	26 do.	
	Tempeft Thornton	5 Mar 1756	
	William Marfhall	28 June	
	James Mansfield	17 Sept. 1757	
Chaplain - -	William Tifdal	25 Aug. 1747	
Adjutant - -	Pelham Maitland	30 Mar. 1754	
Surgeon - -	James Johnfton	10 Nov. 1750	

Agent, Mr. Guerin, Crown-Court, Weftminfter.

Eighth

Rank.	Name.	Rank in the Regiment.	Army.
Colonel	John Waldegrave	22 Jan. 1755	M. Gen. 10 Feb. 57
Lieut Col.	John Severn	20 Feb. 1749-50	Col 7 June 1758
Major	William Lushington	22 Nov. 1756	
Captain	Thomas Hamilton James Monsergh Clement Wolseley	31 Aug. 1747 4 Sept 1754 16 Feb. 1756	8 May 1746
Captain Lieut.	James Graham	15 Feb. 1747-8	
Lieutenant	John Agnew Arthur Johnston Christopher Conyers James Fleming Edward Fitzgerald	31 Aug. 1744 19 Mar 1746-7 7 Apr. 1750 27 Apr. 1756 21 Sept.	
Cornet	Lewis Moore Nathaniel Cook Francis Brook Henry Irwin Richard Jones Edward Wall	20 June 1753 12 Mar. 1754 10 Dec. 1755 27 Apr 1756 do 21 Sept.	
Chaplain	Elias Handcock	21 Sept 1756	
Adjutant	St. George Hatfield	3 June 1752	
Surgeon	Thomas Wetherilt	24 Jan. 1752	

Agent, Mr. Chaigneau, Dublin.

Ninth

Rank	Name	Rank in the	
		Regiment	Army
Colonel - -	Philip Honywood	22 May 1756	17 Mar 1752
Lieut Col -	Oven Wynne	9 Apr. 1756	
Major - -	Edward Clayton	9 Apr. 1756	
Captain - -	John Cullen Henry Clarke Robert French	9 Apr. 1756 22 Nov 3 Nov 1757	
Captain Lieut.	Hugh Moore	22 Nov. 1756	
Lieutenant -	Paul Bush William Leatham James Brown Dixie Coddington Henry Hughes	20 June 1753 9 Apr 1756 22 Nov. 30 July 1737 3 Nov.	
Cornet - -	Richard Saunders Enoch Sterne Robert Waller John Francis Erskine Richard Vandeleur John Adlercron	9 Apr. 1756 27 do. 22 Nov 27 July 1757 30 do. 3 Nov.	26 Feb. 1756
Chaplain - - Adjutant - - Surgeon - -	Maurice Gough Thomas Troboe Henry Man	12 May 1754 do.	

Agent, Mr Waddocke, Dublin.

Tenth

| Rank. | Name. | Rank in the | |
		Regiment.	Army.
Colonel - -	Sir John Mordaunt	1 Nov. 1749	L. Gen. 1 May 54
Lieut. Col. -	Henry Whitley	15 Mar. 47-8	
Major - -	Robert Sloper	28 Dec. 1755	
Captain - -	{ Richard Davenport John Vaughan Samuel Carter Robert Atkinfon	2 Mar 1754 28 Jan. 1755 24 Dec. 25 do.	
Captain Lieut.	Tho. Osb Mordaunt	25 Dec 1755	
Lieutenant -	{ Tho. Strong Hall Peter Renouard Sam Dukenfield Anthony Lovebond William Morrice William Tancred	21 Apr. 1753 28 Jan. 1755 20 Dec 26 do. 23 Mar. 1756 8 Nov.	
Cornet - -	{ John Jones Bodo Knigge Lieu Arthur Fellows Frederick Coldwell Charles Eisfine Richard Brudoe James Foreman	20 Dec. 1755 25 do. 25 do. 26 do. 23 Mar. 1756 2 Sept 8 Nov.	2 Oct. 1755
Chaplain -	Horace Hammond	3 Feb 1741-2	
Adjutant - -	Bodo Knigge	31 May 1755	
Surgeon - -	Thomas Edington	29 Apr. 1757	

Agent, Mr. Calcraft, Channel Row, Westminster.

Eleventh

Rank.	Name	Rank in the	
		Regiment.	Army.
Colonel - -	Wm. E. of Ancram	8 Feb. 1752	L. Gen 27 Jan. 1758
Lieut Col. -	William Gardner	26 June 1754	
Major - -	George Warde	2 June 1756	
Captain - -	Simon Polhill	29 May 1754	
	David Bell	8 Apr. 1755	
	William Lindfay	25 Dec.	
	Salem Philby	8 May 1758	
Captain Lieut.	George Brown	8 May 1758	
Lieutenant -	John Fletcher	26 Dec. 1755	
	Edward Hall	26 July 1756	
	Samuel Birch	17 Sept. 1757	
	Andrew Lyon	26 Jan. 1758	
	Adam Cockburne	10 Feb	
	Hon Wm Gordon	8 May	
Cornet - -	Thomas Paterson	2 Sept. 1756	
	Martin Bafil	3 do	
	Erafmus Phillips	26 Oct. 1757	
	Alex Purves	20 Dec	
	Samuel Ruxton	10 Feb 1758	
	Nehemiah Winter	1 Mar	
	John Jennings	8 May	
Chaplain - -	Duncan Menzies	31 May 1755	
Adjutant - -	Thomas Paterson	21 Jan 1756	
Surgeon - -	John Butler	21 Jan 1756	

Agent, Mr. Rofs, Conduit-ftreet.

Twelfth

Rank.	Name	Rank in the	
		Regiment	Army
Colonel -	Sir J Whitefoord, Bt. 18 Jan. 49-50		M.Gen. 19 Jan. 1758
Lieut. Col.	John Owen	22 Dec. 1747	
Major -	John Wyune	18 Nov. 1755	
Captain -	Robert Mulihallen	11 May 1748	
	Ponfonby Moore	16 Dec 1752	
	William Bury	4 Sept. 1754	
Captain Lieut.	Chudleigh Morgan	22 June 1757	
Lieutenant -	Thomas Tickell	4 Sept. 1754	
	James Beers	22 Jan. 1755	
	Robert Ogle	10 Dec.	16 May 1747
	George Biereton	27 Apr 1756	
	Joseph Walker	22 June 1757	
Cornet -	Robert Bunbury	12 Mar. 1754	
	Hugh Henry	do	
	Wm Pennyfeather	22 Jan. 1755	
	Malcoln Rankin	10 Dec.	
	John Grace	22 June 1757	
	Arthur Usher	27 May 1758	
Chaplain -	Tho Widenham	11 Feb 1758	
Adjutant -	John Siree	3 June 1753	
Surgeon -	James Dudington	11 Feb. 1758	

Agent, Mr. Cockburn, Dublin.

Thirteent's

Rank.	Name	Rank in the	
		Regiment.	Army
Colonel -	John Moftyn	8 July 1754	M. Gen 8 Feb 1757
Lieutenant Col.	James Johnfton	2 Dec 1754	
Major - - -	John Balaguire	23 June 1756	4 Sept. 1754
Captain - -	{ Thomas Crow James Blaquiere John Alcock	19 Sept. 1747 4 Feb 1748-9 10 Dec 1755	
Captain Lieut.	William Tighe	10 Dec 1755	
Lieutenant - -	{ Ambrofe Upton John French John Karr John Ladereze Silvefter Devenifh	24 May 1749 20 Feb. 49-50 10 Dec. 1755 27 Apr 1756 22 June 1757	
Cornet - -	{ Francis Campbell Owen Lindfey John Keily Charles Euftace John Nettles Henry Alcock	4 Sept. 1754 10 Dec. 1755 do 27 Apr. 1756 22 June 1757 27 May 1758	
Chaplain - - -	Peter Pelifier	29 May 1750	
Adjutant - - -	Francis Campbell	3 June 1752	
Surgeon - - -	Owen Lindfey	24 Jun 1752	

Agent, M. Chaigneau, Dublin.

Rank.	Name.	Rank in the	
		Regiment.	Army.
Colonel - -	John Campbell	5 Apr. 1757	10 Nov 1755.
Lieutenant Col.	Thomas Eile	4 Sept. 1754	
Major - -	Marcus Norman	2 Jan 1756	
Captain - -	{ Daniel Chenevix Robert Brown John Forde	4 Sept. 1754 8 Mar. 1757 11 Feb. 1758	
Captain Lieut.	John Mayne	12 Mar. 1754	
Lieutenant -	{ Trevor Smith Thomas Pepper Arthur Molesworth Lewillin Nash Robert Howard	12 Sept. 1745 2 Jan. 1756 9 Apr. 8 Mar. 1757 11 Feb. 1758	
Cornet - -	{ Andrew Jacob T. Wyndh Goddard John Smith James Obrien Grice Blakeney Philip Savage	25 May 1744 22 Apr. 1749 12 Mar. 1754 9 Apr. 1756 8 Mar. 1757 11 Feb. 1758	
Chaplain - -	Peter Vatass		
Adjutant - -	Jeremiah Healy	7 Dec 1756	
Surgeon - -	Thomas Irving	17 Aug. 1747	

Agent, Mr.   Dublin.

First

Rank	Name.	Rank in the	
		Regiment	Army
Colonel - -	John Vifc. Ligonier	30 Nov. 1757	F. Mar. 30 Nov 57
Lieutenant Col.	Alexander Dury	27 Apr. 1749	M. Gen. 4 Feb. 57
Fiift Major - -	Edward Carr	22 Dec. 1753	M. Gen. 21 Feb. 57
Second Major -	James Durand	22 Dec. 1753	Col. 22 Dec. 1753
Captain and Lieut. Colonel	Joseph Hudfon	11 Apr 1746	Col. 24 May 1756
	Edmond Wynne	22 Feb. 1747-8	
	John Seabright	2 May 1749	
	Hon George Carv	23 Nov 1750	
	Hon Wm Keppel	28 Apr. 1751	
	Richard Peirfon	16 Mar 1752	
	Edward Urmfton	23 Nov. 1753	
	Earl of Dalhoufie	22 Dec	
	Septimus Robinfon	29 May 1754	
	John Salter	28 Aug	
	Philip Sheiard	24 Mar 1755	
	George Lane Parker	5 Nov.	
	Nevill Tatton	18 do.	
	Ld Fied Cavendifh	1 June 1756	Col 7 May 1758
	Richard Lambart	5 do.	
	Alexander Maitland	6 do.	
	Hen E. of Pembroke	8 Sept	Col 10 May 1758
	G Ms of Blandford	8 Apr 1758	
	Lancelot Baugh	1 May	
	Rowland Alfton	2 do.	
	William Style	3 do.	
	Charles Hotham	5 do.	25 June 1757
	Henry Clinton	6 do.	
	Charles Fitzroy	9 do.	
Capt. Lt. & Lt. Col	Guy Carleton	18 June 1757	

Lieutenant

Lieut. and Capt.

George Hele Treby 28 Mar 1751
William Tryon   12 Oct.
Thomas Dickens   30 do
Ch. Lewis Mordaunt 16 Mar. 1752
Spencer Cowper   2 Feb 1753
Nathaniel Manlove   7 June
William Miles   11 do.
George Evans   15 Oct.
Edm Knevet Wilſon 26 Nov.
Richard Pownall   27 do.
Edward Craig   28 Aug. 1754
William Thornton   7 Oct.
Thomas Howard   28 Jan. 1755
William Caſtle   25 Mar.
William Hudſon   14 July
Henry Wickham   12 Nov.
Rich Shuckburgh   30 Dec.
George Bridgeman   13 June 1756
John Jones   26 Oct.
Robert Haſelar   16 July 1757
William Amherſt   21 Sept.
John Johnſon   11 Nov.
Samuel Wollaſton   12 do.
Weſt Hyde   19 do
Thomas Cox   10 Feb. 1758
Charles Goldsworthy 6 May
William Fauquier   7 do.
James Walker   8 do.
Thomas Rolt   9 do.
William Fielding   do
Philip De Salis   19 June

18 March 1755

Enſign

	Anthony David	24 Mar 1755	17 Aug. 1752
	E. P. Medows	14 July	
	George Girth	6 Oct.	Lieut. 4 Jan. 1758
	Charles Farnaby	12 Nov	
	Robert Jenkinson	26 do	15 Oct 1754
	George Evelyn	14 Jan. 1756	
	Ridgway Owen Merrick	20 Mar	27 Dec 1755
	John Howard	13 June	
	Sir Al. Gilmour, Bt	14 do.	
	Charles Dering	5 Sept.	
	William Wilson	26 Oct	
	Ch. Lord Brome	8 Dec.	
Ensign	Rich. John Powis	16 July 1757	9 Apr. 1756
	St. John Jefferys	21 Sept.	
	John Cocks	11 Nov.	
	Temple West	12 do.	
	Mordaunt Martin	19 do	
	Thomas Middleton	10 Feb 1758.	
	Thomas Edmondes	8 May	
	Gerrard Lake	9 do.	
	John Bartlet Allen	10 do.	
	Edward Goat	23 do	
	Michael Cox	19 June	
	Charles Cotterell		27 Dec. 1755

Chaplain	Richard Buckendon	27 May 1751
Adjutant	William Hudson	18 June 1753
	Richard Pownall	12 May 1753
	William Amherst	26 Nov. 1755
Quarter Master	Rice Williams	1 May 1745
Surgeon	Lewis Davies	18 Apr. 1743
Sollicitor	William Luard	19 Nov. 1757

Agent, Mr. Cox, Albemarle-ftreet.

Coldstream

		Rank in the	
Rank.	*Name.*	*Regiment*	*Army.*
Colonel - -	James, Ld. Tyrawly	8 Apr. 1755	Lt. Gen. 31 Mar. 43
Lieutenant Col.	Bennet Noel	22 Dec. 1755	M. Gen. 26 Jan. 58
First Major -	Julius Cæsar	25 Dec. 1755	Col. 12 May 1753
Second Major	William A'Court	29 Dec. 1755	Col. 29 Dec 1755
Captain and Lieut Colonel	John Thomas	17 Feb 1747-8	
	William Ganfell	28 Nov. 1749	
	Charles Craig	30 Jan. 1750-1	
	John Robinson	15 Mar 1752	
	John Clavering	23 Dec.	
	Hon Chad. Drayncy	8 June 1753	
	Charles Vernon	10 do.	
	William Evelyn	27 Aug. 1754	
	Martin Sandys	25 Mar. 1755	
	Ruvigny De Cosne	4 Nov.	
	George Bodens	1 Jan. 1756	
	William Sorell	4 June	
	Francis Craig	28 Apr. 1758	
	Henry Lister	4 May	
Capt. Lt &Lt.Col.	John Burgoyne	10 May 1758	
Lieut & Captain	Sir W. Wiseman, Bt.	5 Apr. 1748	
	Thomas Clarke	15 May 1749	27 Sept. 1745
	Charles Ramsford	30 Jan. 1750-1	
	William Wright	30 Apr 1751	14 July 1749
	Edward Mathews	17 Dec.	
	Henry Trelawny	4 Mar. 1752	
	William Gwyn	16 do.	

Lieutenant

Lieut. & Captain	James Craig	23 Dec. 1752
	Thomas d'Avenant	12 June 1753
	John Thornton	24 July 1754
	William Winch	27 Aug.
	Lewis Buckeridge	14 July 1755
	Anth Geo. Martin	13 Jan. 1756
	Charles O'Hara	14 do.
	George Scott	12 June
	Timothy C ſwall	27 Oct.
	Richard Huſſey	2 May 1758
	Wadham Wyndham	3 do.
	Wm. Charles Sloper	4 do.

Enſign	Geo. Auguſt. Wyvill	24 July 1754	10 Nov 1750
	William Schutz	28 Aug	
	Charles Morgan	4 Oct 1755	
	Thomas Biſhop	13 Jan 1756	
	Mathew Smith	23 Mar.	
	John Lambton	12 June	8 Aug. 1755
	Henry Dilkes	21 do.	
	George Banks	6 Sept.	
	William Woſeley	2 Sept. 1757	
	John Twiſleton	3 do.	
	George Morgan	1 Mar 1758	2 Sept 1756
	Robert Eden	8 May	4 Feb. 1757
	James Birch	9 do.	
	William Bowyer	10 do.	
	Lewis George Dive	11 do.	
	John Edmondes	23 do.	

Chaplain	John Jeffreys	11 May 1742
Adjutant	Thomas d'Avenant	21 Dec 1746
	Charles Ransford	8 Apr. 1758
Quarter Maſter	William Wright	30 Apr. 1751
Surgeon	Peter Tuquet	19 Jan. 1746-7
Sollicitor	Gilbert Elliott	2 June 1744

Agent Mr. Fiſher, Axe-Yard, Weſtminſter.

Rank.	Name	Rank in the	
		Regiment.	Army.
Colonel - -	John Earl of Rothes	29 Apr 1752	Lt. Gen. 5 Aug 47
Lieutenant Col.	Andrew Robinson	2 May 1758	Col. 24 Dec. 1755
First Major -	John Griffin Griffin	2 May 1758	Col 29 May 1756
Second Major	John Prideaux	2 May 1758	Col. 2 May 1758
Captain and Lieut. Colonel	Thomas Burges John Gore John Furbar James Forrester John Wells Manfoe Frederick Montage. Blomer John Scott Lord Adam Gordon Robert Campbell Wm Cuninghame Hon Rob. Brudenell Mackpherson Neale William Williams	28 Apr. 1749 11 Apr 1750 29 Jan 1750-1 4 Mar. 9 June 1753 11 do. 27 Aug. 31 Dec. 1755 2 Jan. 1756 3 June 7 May 1757 31 Jan. 1758 7 Apr 29 do.	
Cap Lt & Lt.Col.	Bernard Hyde	30 Apr 1758	
Lieut. & Captain	Seth Robinson William Witthed Michael Hudson Daniel Jones	9 Mar 1746-7 16 Feb 1747-8 - Aug. 1749 21 Feb 49-50	

Lieutenant

Lieut. & Captain	John Smith	27 Aug 1753	
	George Tash	6 Oct.	
	T. More Mollineaux	23 Nov.	
	William Wynyard	30 Mar 1754	
	John Neale	23 Aug 1755	
	John E. of Dunmore	5 Nov.	
	Nathaniel Gould	11 June 1756	
	George Osborne	19 Feb. 1757	
	William Faucitt	1 Mar.	
	Fred. Hollingsworth	2 Oct.	8 Mar. 1757
	William Kingsley	12 Nov.	
	John Cathcart	7 Apr. 1758	
	Rd. Bempde Johnson	5 May	
	Thomas Twisleton	8 do.	
	James Douglas	5 June	5 Sept 1756

Ensign	Humphry Stevens	31 Mar 1755	
	Francis Twisleton	23 Aug.	
	Alexand. Campbell	5 Oct	
	H. Cosmo Gordon	15 Jan. 1756	
	Arthur Owen	22 do.	
	Hon. Geo. Forbes	20 June	
	Edw. Bayntun Rolt	3 Sept.	
	Charles Madan	4 do.	15 Jan. 1756
	Thomas Needham	7 do.	
	John Pennington	17 Dec.	
	Francis Hall	19 Feb 1757	
	Roderick Gwynne	14 May	
	Thomas Byron	12 Nov	
	Henry Northcote	7 Apr. 1758	
	Sir John Chisham Bt	8 May	
	James Hope	9 do.	

Chaplain	George Bruce	31 Jan. 1756
Adjutant	Michael Hudson	17 May 1751
	William Faucitt	1 Dec 1757
Quarter Master	John Colladon	28 May 1752
Surgeon	William Fordyce	26 Dec. 1750
Sollicitor	George Ross	26 May 1747

Agent, Mr. Ross. Conduit-street.

Rank.	Name.	Rank in the Battalion	Army.
Colonel - -	James St. Clair	27 June 1737	Lt. Gen 4 June 45
Lieutenant Col.	Rt.Dal HornElphinston	20 June 1753	
Major - -	David Lindsay	27 May 1758	
Captain - -	John Curringham	1 Apr. 1744	
	James Edmonston	11 June	
	John Nairn	1 May 1745	
	James Cunningham	3 June 1752	
	James Masterton	22 Jan 1757	
	George Agnew	16 Feb. 1756	
	Benj. Mainwaring	2 Feb. 175	
Captain Lieut.	James Spittall	7 May 1757	
Lieutenant - -	Abraham Stewart	16 Feb. 1756	
	Thomas Frazer	9 Apr.	
	Alexander Joass	27 do	
	Peter Bradstreet	21 Sept.	
	Duncan Urquhart	do.	
	Charles Congelton	22 Nov.	
	Alexander Gordon	do.	
	Pointz Stewart	do.	
	Henry Balfour Jun.	2 Feb. 1757	
	Maximilian Faviere	7 May	
Ensign - -	Samuel Stevenson	27 Apr. 1756	
	Arthur Gore	21 Sept.	
	James Stuart	22 Nov.	
	Oliver Nicolls	do.	
	James Lumisden	2 Feb. 1757	
	John Barber	do.	
	William Le Hunt	do.	
	John Duddingston	do.	
	Tho. Woollacombe	7 May	
Chaplain	Alexander Logie	14 June 1746	
Adjutant	Thomas Frazer	16 Nov 1756	
Surgeon	Theodore Forbes	10 Dec. 1755	

Agent, Capt. Montgomery, Dublin.

First

Rank.	Name.	Rank in the Battalion.	Rank in the Army.
Colonel - -	Lt. Gen. Ja St Clair		
Lieut. Colonel	William Forster	24 Dec. 1755	
Major - -	Frederick Hamilton	7 May 1757	
Captain - -	Robert Mirrie	25 June 1747	7 Jan. 1747-8
	Alexander Hay	12 Mar. 1754	
	James Roberton	4 Sept.	
	Patrick Gordon	16 Feb. 1756	
	James Wall	do.	
	Benjamin Gordon	2 Feb. 1757	
	Robert Wilmot	25 do.	
	John Abercrombie	7 May	
Lieutenant -	William Cockburn	22 Jan 1755	
	Henry Balfour	15 Mar.	
	Charles Forbes	15 Feb. 1756	
	James Fenton	do.	
	John Hill	9 Apr.	
	James Douglass	27 do.	
	John Knox	21 Sept.	
	John Gordon	22 Nov.	
	Dudley Ashe	do.	
	Robert M'Kinen	25 Dec.	19 Sept. 1745
	Josiah How	26 do.	15 Sept. 1754
	Francis Fitzsimons	27 do.	16 do.
	Thomas Moncriffe	28 do.	do.
	James M'Manus	29 do.	18 do.
	Trevor Newland	30 do.	22 Oct. 1755
	Archibald Hamilton	31 do.	24 do.
	William Cook	1 Jan. 1757	25 do.
	Adolphus Benzell	2 do.	24 Nov.
	Alexander Baillie	2 Feb.	
	James Stuart	do.	
	Richard Marshall	25 do.	
Ensign - -	Patrick West	27 Apr. 1756	
	Henry Marcell	do	
	Robert Cook	do.	
	George Burton	do.	
	Henry Waterson	22 Nov	
	Thomas Roth	2 Feb 1757	
	John Baggs	do.	
	Richard Frend	do.	
	James Eddingstone	2 Mar.	
Chaplain - -	Wm. Halliburton	22 May 1747	
Adjutant - -	Henry Balfour	25 Feb. 1757	
Quarter Master	James Douglas	19 Feb. 1757	
Surgeon - -	John M'Colme	1 May 1744	

Agent, Mr. Wilson, Craven-Street, the Strand.

Rank.	Name	Rank in the Regiment.	Army.
Colonel - -	John Fitz William	12 Nov. 1755	
Lieut. Colonel	James Molefworth	22 Nov. 1756	
Major - -	Edward Windus	22 Nov. 1756	
Captain - -	John Morris George Alexander Hudfon Bernard Peter Labilliere Robert Raitt Thomas Simes Michael Nickfon	20 June 1753 10 Dec. 1755 16 Feb. 1756 do. 22 Nov. 8 Mar. 1757 7 May	3 Sept. 1747
Captain Lieut.	Hugh Bailey	7 May 1757	
Lieutenant -	John Barker Robert Donkin Ifaac Haman Peter Dambon Henry Shaw George Ford Samuel Molcher Charles Baldwin John Jackfon Henry Flood	20 June 1753 4 Sept. 1754 10 Dec. 1755 27 Apr. 1756 do. do. 21 Sept. 22 Nov. 8 Mar. 1757 7 May	
Enfign - -	Bernard Shaw William Evans Richard Phillips William Gray Richard Campbell Ezek. Davis Duncan Avarel Daniel James Ball William Glafcott	27 Apr. 1756 do. do. do. 16 Nov. 27 do. 4 Jan. 1757 8 Mar. 7 May	
Chaplain - -	John Achmuty	22 Feb 1741	
Adjutant - -	John Jackfon	21 Sept. 1756	
Surgeon - -	Geo. Majoribanks	18 Apr. 1745	

Agent, Mr. Defbrifay, Dublin.

Third

Rank	Name.	Rank in the Regiment	Army.
Colonel - -	George Howard	21 Aug 1749	M. Gen. 16 Jan. 58
Lieut. Colonel	Cyrus Trapaud	15 Feb. 1749-50	
Major - -	Shackburgh Hewett	3 Sept 1756	
Captain - -	Roger Townſhend	28 June 1751	Lt. Col 1 Feb 1758
	Lamund Imber	21 Mar. 1753	3 Mar. 1747-8
	James Johnſton	10 Oct 1755	
	John Biddulph	15 June 1756	
	Thomas Mc Leroth	26 Aug.	22 Mar 1747-8
	Thomas Bunbury	28 do	
	George Nicholſon	29 do.	
	William Stiell	30 do.	
Captain Lieut.	Thomas Dawſon	9 Mar 1757	
Lieutenant -	George Acklom	3 Oct. 1755	
	Joſeph Fenton	31 Mar. 1756	
	Thomas Muſgrave	21 June	
	Alex. Donaldſon	25 Aug.	27 Apr. 1756
	Robert Home	28 do.	
	Scipio Carnac	29 do.	
	William Felton	30 do	
	Thomas Ferguſon	31 do.	
	James Bramham	1 Sept	Capt. 14 May 1757
	Robert Tullidelph	2 do.	
	John Hillary	3 do.	
	Charles Campbell	9 Mar. 1757	
	Francis Baille	21 Sept.	23 Oct. 1755
	James Bradſhaw	22 do	24 Oct. 1755
	David Honywood	25 do.	
	Thomas Da Coſta	26 do.	
	William Spry	27 do.	
	Alexander Paterſon	29 do.	
Enſign - - -	John Johnſton	2 Sept. 1756	
	Robert Grier	4 do.	
	Tho. Woods Knollis	9 Mar. 1757	
	John Greenwood	24 Sept	
	Nathaniel Philips	25 do.	
	Geo Armand Powlett	26 do.	
	John Nodes	28 do.	
	John Hamilton	19 June 1758	
Chaplain - -	George Carr	24 Nov 1753	
Adjutant - -	Thomas Ferguſon	1 May 1745	
Quarter Maſter	Samuel Gay	25 Aug. 1750	
Surgeon - -	Abraham Gordon	11 Oct 1746	

Agent, Mr Guerin, Crown-Court, Weſtminſter.

Fourth

Rank.	Name.	Regiment.	Army.
		Rank in the	
Colonel - -	Alex. Duroure	12 May 1756	M. Gen. 24 Jan. 58
Lieut. Colonel	Byam Crump	17 Dec. 1757	29 Dec. 1755
Major - -	Thomas Hardy	11 Jan. 1756	
Captain - -	Jonas Thompson	22 July 1751	
	Joseph Partridge	13 Oct. 1755	
	Thomas Cooke	11 Jan. 1756	
	Thomas Ogle	26 Aug.	27 Apr. 1756
	Colin Campbell	27 do.	27 Apr. 1756
	George Kennedy	28 do.	
	James Campbell	29 do	
	Humphry Bland	3 Sept.	
Captain Lieut.	Alexander Kennedy	25 Aug. 1756	
Lieutenant -	John Charlton	2 Mar. 1754	
	John Roche	13 Oct. 1755	
	William Abbot	15 do.	
	James Boorder	26 Feb. 1756	
	Tong Wekett	23 Mar.	
	Robert Doriell	24 Aug.	
	Robert Soulby	25 do.	12 May 1753
	James Leslie	27 do.	27 April 1756
	James Winchester	28 do.	
	William Henderson	30 do.	
	Solomon Milward	1 Sept.	
	Francis Gray	3 do.	
	Simon Mackenzie	27 Jan. 1757	
	George Montgarret	21 Sept.	25 October 1755
	W. Rd. Middlemore	22 do.	18 May 1756
	Gabriel Lewis	25 do.	
	James Welborn	26 do.	
	James Ogilvie	20 Dec.	
Ensign - -	Josiah Martin	17 Dec. 1756	
	Samuel Bullock	6 May 1757	
	Robert Paul	24 Sept.	
	William Sellwood	25 do	
	William Cosby	26 do.	
	Walter Home	28 do.	
	Geo. Harry Chitty	29 do.	
	John Bicford	26 Mar. 1758	
Chaplain, - -	John Duncan	2 May 1745	
Adjutant - -	Robert Dorrell	24 July 1747	
Quarter Master	William Sellwood	25 Aug. 1756	
Surgeon - -	William Everard	17 Dec. 1754	

Agent, Mr. Wiseman, King-Street, St. Anns.

Fifth

Rank.	Name.	Rank in the Regiment.	Army.
Colonel - -	Ld. Geo. Bentinck	20 Aug. 1754	3 March 1752
Lieut. Colonel	John Irwin	27 Nov. 1752	
Major - -	William Euftace	17 Nov. 1757	
Captain - -	George Rawfon	9 Feb 1750-1	
	James Nugent	24 Jan. 1752	
	Charles Heathcote	4 Sept. 1754	
	David Rofs	1 Oct. 1755	
	Whitfhed Keene	4 Mar 1756	
	Henry Townfhend	8 May 1758	
Captain Lieut.	Bernard Higgins	8 May 1758	
Lieutenant	James Bromhead	22 Jan. 1755	
	James Smith	1 Oct	
	Bennet Cuthbertfon	2 do.	
	Franklin Kerby	4 Mar. 1756	
	Daniel Rea	29 Aug.	
	Edward Webb	30 do.	
	Richard Davis	31 do.	
	Robert Shearing	2 Sept.	
	Robert Littlewood	22 Apr 1757	
	James Nairne	23 Sept.	
	James Davis	24 do.	
	Adam Williamfon	25 do.	
	John Bonner	27 do.	
	John Smith	28 do.	
	John Baillie	29 do.	
	John Grey	30 do	
	John Watts Parker	8 May 1758	
	Chriftopher Cooper	Aug.	
Enfign - -	William Sleigh	8 July 1757	
	Benjamin Baker	2 Oct.	
	Gilbert Warman	3 do.	
	Anthony Nugent	4 do.	
	Henry Downe	5 do.	
	Robert Palmer	6 do.	
	Thomas Robinfon	23 May 1758	
	Richard Temple	Aug.	
Chaplain - -	Eth. Powell Wogan	18 June 1757	
Adjutant - -	Bennet Cuthbertfon	23 Aug 1755	
Quarter Mafter	James Smith	12 Mar. 1755	
Surgeon - -	James Inglis	26 Oct 1757	

Agent, Mr. Calcraft, Channel-Row, Weftminfter.

Sixth

Rank.	Name.	Rank in the	
		Regiment.	Army.
Colonel - -	John Guife	1 Nov. 1738	L. Gen. 7 June 45
Lieut. Colonel	Robert Scott	8 Jan. 1756	
Major - - -	Sir Hugh Williams, Bt.	10 Jan. 1756	
Captain - -	⎧ John Swettenham ⎪ Henry Patton ⎪ Henry Yeo Taaffe ⎨ Jacob Moody ⎪ George Forfter ⎪ Hamlet Wade ⎩ John Maxwell	16 Mar. 1741-2 30 Sept. 1746 16 Jan. 49-50 23 Dec. 1752 21 Mar. 1753 9 April 1754 3 Aug. 1757	
Captain Lieut.	Mathew Derenzy	3 Aug. 1757	
Lieutenant -	⎧ Miller Hill Hunt ⎪ Folliot Whiteway ⎪ Robert Cay ⎪ James Patton ⎨ John Guife ⎪ James Batchelor ⎪ James Somerville ⎪ William Brabazon ⎪ Thomas Cole ⎩ John Dale	30 Sept. 1746 27 Nov. 1752 21 Mar. 1753 9 Apr. 1754 8 Apr. 1755 5 Nov. 27 Dec. 30 Aug. 1756 2 Sept. 3 Aug. 1757	
Enfign - -	⎧ James Barnes ⎪ Thomas Maude ⎪ Joseph Hamilton ⎪ Thomas Dobyns ⎨ Thomas Munn ⎪ Lachlan Leflie ⎪ Thomas Browne ⎪ Zachariah Moore ⎩ William Hurft	8 Apr. 1755 18 June 5 Nov. 3 Sept. 1756 4 Oct. 1757 1 Dec. 19 June 1758 20 do. Aug.	25 Mar. 1758
Chaplain - -	John Mawer	9 Aug. 1756	
Adjutant - -	Miller Hill Hunt	13 May 1754	
Quarter Mafter	John Guife	7 Oct. 1756	
Surgeon - -	James Stewart	17 Aug. 1753	

Agent, Mr. Winter, Brewer-ftreet.

Seventh

Rank.	Name.	Rank in the Regiment.	Army.
Colonel -	Lord Robert Bertie	20 Aug. 1754	4 Mar. 1752
Lieut. Colonel	Marcus Smith	3 June 1752	
Major -	Henry Gore	30 Dec. 1755	
Captain -	Thomas Gwilliam	2 May 1751	
	James Edgar	20 June 1753	
	Moses Corbett	22 Jan. 1755	
	James Harvey	15 Oct.	
	John Caldwell	20 Dec.	
	Patrick Drumgole	29 July 1757	
	Thomas Shears	8 May 1758	
Captain Lieut.	Edward Brice Dobbs	8 May 1758	
Lieutenant -	John Conyngham	16 Dec. 1752	
	Philip Despard	4 Sept. 1754	
	Ralph Donnellan	24 Apr. 1755	
	Francis Kinneer	2 Oct.	
	James Gardner	5 do.	
	Timothy Newmarsh	30 Dec.	
	Sheringt. Davenport	11 Feb. 1756	
	William Dundas	25 Aug.	
	Joseph Sisson	29 do.	
	Benjamin Johnson	30 do.	
	William Howard	17 Dec.	
	Charles Ward	12 Jan. 1757	
	John Strode	13 Feb.	
	Henry Tracey	do.	
	Jonas Jeffery Avarne	29 Apr.	
	John Gilpin Sawrey	8 July	
	Thomas Tennison	29 do.	
	Apollos Morris	8 May 1758	
	Frederick Disney	19 June	
Chaplain -	Edmund Baxter	4 Sept. 1738	
Adjutant -	Moses Corbett	27 Nov. 1752	
Quarter Master	Ralph Donnellan	19 Feb. 1757	
Surgeon -	John Fryer	4 Jan. 1749-50	

Agent, Mr. Calcraft, Channel-Row, Westminster.

H

Eighth

Rank.	Name.	Rank in the Regiment.	Rank in the Army.
Colonel - -	Edward Wolfe	25 Apr. 1745	L. Gen. 20 Sept. 47
Lieut. Colonel	John La Faussille	27 Apr. 1749	
Major - -	John Cook	4 Sept. 1756	
Captain - -	Henry Boisragon	22 Apr. 1752	
	Francis Wilkinson	27 Aug. 1753	
	John Corrance	26 Feb. 1755	
	Tho. Spencer Wilson	16 Oct.	
	James Webb	2 Nov	
	James Dundass	25 Aug. 1756	18 Apr. 1747
	Obadiah Bourne	27 do.	27 Apr. 1756
Captain Lieut.	Henry Lee	25 Aug. 1756	
Lieutenant	Thomas Backhouse	27 Aug. 1753	
	Thomas Stewart	31 May	
	Robert Spence	1 Oct.	10 Sept. 1746
	Grant Scott	2 do.	
	Christopher Brown	4 do.	
	Ebenezer Warren	25 Aug. 1756	18 Jan. 1756
	Solgard Marshall	26 do.	23 June 1756
	John Young	27 do.	
	Rich. Berr Lernoult	29 do.	
	Richard Dudgeon	1 Sept.	Capt. Lt. 4 Jan. 58
	Arent Schuyler De Peister	21 Sept. 1757	10 June 1756
	Theophilus Dame	22 do.	11 June 1756
	Augustus Alt	25 do.	
	George Forster	26 do.	
	Mungo Law	28 do.	
	Dick Culhford	29 do.	
	William Morrison	30 do.	
	Mitchelbourne Knox	3 Oct.	
Ensign - -	Roger Parke	5 Apr. 1757	
	Edmund Boyle	24 Sept.	
	Henry Savage	26 do.	
	Benjamin Ashe	28 do.	
	Charles Parke	30 do.	
	Roger Twigge	1 Oct.	
	Richard Taylor	2 do.	
	William Marler	6 do.	
Chaplain - -	George Hatfield	5 Aug. 1747	
Adjutant - -	Henry Lee	29 Oct. 1754	
Quarter Master	Grant Scott	28 June 1756	
Surgeon - -	Robert Miller	13 Sept. 1745	

Agent, Mr. Fisher, Axe-Yard, Westminster.

Ninth

Rank.	Name.	Rank in the Regiment	Army.
Colonel - -	Hon. Joseph Yorke	18 Mar. 1755	M. Gen. 18 Jan 58
Lieut. Colonel	Richard Worge	4 Oct. 1754	
Major - -	Hans Musgrave	12 Jan. 1758	
Captain - -	Phin John Edgar	19 June 1751	
	Francis Ogilvie	20 June 1753	
	John Dalrymple	do.	
	Alexander Wilkie	22 Jan. 1755	
	George Godfrey	14 Oct.	
	James Dalrymple	13 Nov.	
	Lawrence Reynolds	12 Jan. 1758	
Captain Lieut.	John Harris	28 Aug. 1756	
Lieutenant -	Peter Aylward	20 June 1753	
	Robert Eyre	22 Jan. 1755	
	Mason Bolton	2 Oct.	
	Nicholas Nugent	11 Feb. 1756	
	Arthur Beard	28 Aug.	
	Andrew Rainsford	1 Sept.	
	Robert Edmeson	18 Jan. 1757	
	Samuel Surman	12 Jan 1758	
	George Collins	do.	
	James Pampillone	27 May	
Ensign - -	Nich Delacherois	18 May 1756	
	Gabriel Hamilton	14 June	
	Eusebius Chute	28 Aug.	
	Thomas Lewis	1 Sept.	
	Joseph Fish	12 Jan. 1758	
	William Ewer	do.	
	John Gordon	do.	
	George Gill	11 Feb.	
	Samuel Waller	27 May	
Chaplain - -	John Woodroffe	27 July 1757	
Adjutant - -	William Sharpe	20 Nov. 1756	
Surgeon - -	Alexander Shearer	5 Jan. 1750-1	

Agent, Mr. Chaigneau, Dublin.

		Rank in the	
Rank.	Name.	Regiment.	Army.
Colonel - -	Edward Pole	10 Aug. 1749	M. Gen. 9 Feb. 57
Lieut. Colonel	James Gifborne	18 Nov. 1755	
Major - -	Edmund Bradfhaw	23 June 1756	
Captain - -	Francis Smith	23 June 1747	29 Nov 1745
	Benjamin Blackerby	16 Dec. 1752	
	Charles Vallancy	10 Dec. 1755	
	Thomas Wills	do.	
	James Hamilton	27 Apr. 1756	
	William Percival	22 Nov.	
	Henry Baffett	7 May 1757	
Captain Lieut.	Charles Sailly	22 Nov. 1756	
Lieutenant -	Ifrael Mitchell	2 May 1751	13 Dec. 1745
	John Vatafs	12 Mar. 1754	
	Samuel Brown	22 Apr. 1755	
	Mundy Pole	10 Dec.	
	Higate Boyd	do.	
	Robert Dalway	do.	
	Jofeph Sirr	16 Feb. 1756	
	John Hollingworth	27 April	
	Nicholas Gay	8 Mar. 1757	
	Thomas Skeen	7 May	
Enfign - -	William Candler	27 Apr. 1756	
	Thomas Herbert	do.	
	Richard Luther	do.	
	Arthur Hill Brice	do.	
	George Tompkins	do.	
	Aaron Lilly	22 Nov.	
	Jofhua Johnfton	do.	
	Walter Cuffe	8 Mar. 1757	
	Fitzgerald	7 May	
Chaplain - -	Nicholas Hamilton	10 Dec. 1755	
Adjutant - -	Richard Withers	27 Aug. 1757	
Surgeon - -	John Garnet	10 Dec. 1755	

Agent, Mr. Whitlocke, Dublin.

Eleventh

| Rank. | Name. | Rank in the | |
		Regiment.	Army.
Colonel - -	Maurice Bocland	1 Dec. 1747	Lt. Gen. 23 Jan. 58
Lieut. Col. -	Cecil Forrefter	30 Dec. 1755	24 Jan. 1752.
Major - -	Cholmeley Scott	30 Aug 1756	
Captain - -	Robert Welfh	26 Dec. 1750	
	Benjamin Benby	6 Oct. 1755	
	George Robinfon	21 Jan. 1756	
	Robert Trevor	4 June	
	George Maddifon	5 do.	20 Mar. 1755
	Richard Carr	26 Aug.	27 Apr. 1756
	Hugh Sempil	15 July 1758	
Captain Lieut.	Thomas Thorp	15 July 1758	
Lieutenant -	Benjamin Edwards	8 Apr. 1755	
	William Smith	1 Oct.	
	Thomas Gordon	9 Dec.	
	Charles Wingfield	21 Jan. 1756	
	Robert Chefshyre	31 Mar.	
	Robert Rookfby	4 June	
	Thomas Falkner	25 Aug.	27 April 1756
	James Dalton	28 do.	
	Jofeph Thompfon	30 Aug.	
	Ifaac Antrobus	31 do.	
	Luke Sterling	5 Sept.	
	Thomas Elrington	22 do.	25 Aug. 1748
	Henry Nairne	25 do.	
	James Peters	26 do.	
	Edward Ord	27 do.	
	Adam Price	28 do.	
	William Mackenzie	29 do.	
	George Fenwick	15 July 1758	
Enfign - -	Thomas Hope	25 Sept. 1757	
	George Dawes	26 do.	
	John Sutherland	29 do.	
	Benjamin Rogerfon	30 do.	
	Luke Hudfon	1 Oct.	
	PaulDouglasRobertfon	4 do.	
	Wrey J'ans	6 do.	
	William Stephenfon	15 July 1758	
Chaplain - -	Samuel Speed	5 Apr. 1757	
Adjutant - -	Jofeph Thompfon	26 Nov. 1755	
Quarter Mafter	Thomas Gordon	23 Mar. 1756	
Surgeon - -	William Ferguffon	10 May 1751	

Agent, Mr. Winter, Brewer-ftreet.

Twelfth

Rank.	Name.	Regiment.	Army.
			Rank in the
Colonel - -	Robert Napier	22 Apr. 1757	M. Gen. 4 Feb. 56
Lieut Colonel	Wilham Robinfon	10 Nov. 1755	
Major - -	Corbet Parry	6 Sept. 1756	
Captain - -	Peter Chabbert	25 Dec. 1748	
	Robert Ackland	19 Jan. 1748-9	17 July 1747
	Patrick Ogilvie	8 Oct. 1755	
	Thomas Brereton	24 do.	
	Mathias Murray	4 Nov.	
	William Picton	25 Aug. 1756	17 March 1755
	William Cloudefley	26 do.	27 Apr. 1756
Captain Lieut.	Peter Campbell	25 Aug. 1756	
Lieutenant -	Peter Dunbar	8 Apr. 1755	
	WilliamFolkingham	do.	
	Edward Freeman	1 Oct.	
	William Armftrong	3 do.	
	Geo. Tho. Maffey	28 Aug. 1756	
	Philip Stapleton	29 do.	
	George Rofe	31 do.	
	Thomas Lawlefs	1 Sept.	
	George Townfhend	3 do.	
	William Barlow	4 do.	
	Thomas Fletcher	9 Mar. 1757	
	Hugh Montgomery	5 Apr.	
	John Campbell	6 do.	
	Jofeph Walworth	13 May	
	Robert Geo. Bruce	14 do.	
	Thomas Tutterdge	21 Sept.	26 June 1754
	John Crozier	22 do.	
	Robert Lumfdaine	1 July 1758	
Enfign - -	William Green	9 Mar. 1757	
	John Ant. Vazielle	22 do.	
	William Compton	14 May	
	Henry Probyn	3 Oct.	
	John Forbes	4 do.	
	Thomas Trigge	6 do.	
	David Parkhill	1 July 1758	
Chaplain - -	Tho. Milward Key	26 Oct. 1757	
Adjutant - -	Thomas Lawlefs	19 Nov. 1748	
Quarter Mafter	Wm. Folkingham	9 Mar. 1757	
Surgeon - -	William Haftie	19 June 1752	

Agent, Mr. Adair, Pall-mall.

Thirteenth

Rank.	Name.	Rank in the	
		Regiment	Army.
Colonel - -	Harry Pulteney	5 July 1739	L Gen. 8 Aug 1747
Lieut. Col. -	John Craufurd	9 Oct 1749	
Major - -	David Chapeau	5 Apr. 1757	
Captain - -	George M'Kenzie	6 Sept. 1744	
	Samuel Edhoufe	28 June 1746	
	William Jones	9 Oct 1749	12 Jan 1746-7
	Thomas Briftow	11 June 1753	29 May 1747
	David Ogilvy	25 Dec. 1755	
	James Garnham	5 Apr. 1757	
	Hon —— Cornwallis	5 June 1758	
Captain Lieut.	William Moore	5 June 1758	
Lieutenant -	Richard Scudamore	7 Oct. 1754	
	Andrew Edhoufe	7 Oct. 1755	
	Charles Craufurd	29 Dec.	
	Randolph Carleill	30 do.	
	Henry Pu'leine	2 Jan. 1756	
	John Brathwaite	22 Mar.	
	John Raleigh	22 Mar. 1757	
	Edward Townfhend	5 Apr.	
	George Mohun	6 do.	
	Gwynne Wynne	5 June 1758	
Enfign - -	Henry Dalway	2 Jan. 1756	
	Wm. Bannatine	3 do.	
	Bulleine Fancourt	22 Mar	
	George Henderfon	26 Aug.	
	Ducarroll	1 Sept.	
	John Phipps	5 Apr.	Lieut. 4 Jan. 1758
	Pryfe Donaldfon	7 May	
	Hugh Meyrick	7 Mar 1758	17 Sept. 1757
Chaplain -	Samuel Phipps	5 May 1747	
Adjutant -	John Brathwaite	7 Oct 1756	
Quarter Mafter	William Mifon	2 July 1747	
Surgeon - -	John Miller	1 July 1758	

Agent, Mr. Calcraft, Channel-Row, Weftminfter

Fourteenth

		Regiment.	Rank in the Army.
Rank.	Name.		
Colonel -	Charles Jefferyes	7 Sept 1756	3 Jan 1756
Lieut. Col.	Thomas Lister	5 Apr. 1757	
Major -	John Bell	13 Dec. 1755	
Captain -	Edward Booth	1 Aug. 1744	
	John Meard	do.	
	Bartholom Corneille	23 Apr. 1746	
	Thomas Bowyer	do.	
	Jonathan Furlong	2 Mar. 1750-1	
	Geo James Bruere	14 Oct. 1755	
	Lucius Ferd. Cary	26 Dec.	
Captain Lieut.	Thomas Baylies	26 Dec. 1755	
Lieutenant -	James Montresor	23 July 1757	Lt. Col. 4 Jan. 58
	Francis Lind	22 June 1745	
	Thomas Brisbane	8 Apr. 1755	
	Conoly Ball	26 Dec.	
	James Vipond	27 do.	
	Herbert Whitfield	29 do.	
	John Geathin	17 May 1756	
	James Ross	18 do.	
	Peter Ruffell	8 May 1758	
	Charles Cooper	5 June	
Enfign -	William Blackett	5 July 1755	
	Samuel Lindsay	12 Nov.	
	John Dade	3 Jan. 1756	
	Goldfinch	17 May	
	John Jones	18 do.	
	Wm Kitchingham	14 June	
	John Kendall	26 Jan. 1758	
	Wharton Emerson	8 May	
	Edward Fitzgerald	5 June	
Chaplain - -	Hugh Palmer	17 Dec, 1756	
Adjutant - -	Herbert Whitfield	13 Feb. 1757	
Quarter Mafter	Bruere	4 Jan. 1757	
Surgeon - -	Francis Lind	3 June 1726	

Agent, Mr. Calcraft, Channel-Row, Weftminfter.

Fifteenth

Rank.	Name.	Rank in the	
		Regiment.	Army
Colonel - -	Jeffery Amherst	22 May 1756	
Lieut. Colonel	Hon. James Murray	5 Jan 1750-51	
Major - -	William Farquhar	12 Mar. 1754	
Captain - -	Paulus Æmil. Irving	20 June 1753	
	Hect Theo Cramaké	12 Mar. 1754	
	Arthur Loftus	do.	
	Christopher Usher	4 Sept	
	Robert Prescott	22 Jan. 1755	
	James Barbutt	11 Oct	
	Hervey Smyth	8 Nov. 1756	
Captain Lieut.	Manly Williams	29 Aug. 1756	
Lieutenant -	Colin Campbell	4 Sept 1754	
	Samuel Rutherford	do.	
	Patrick Dunbar	22 Jan. 1755	
	Theophilus Paske	1 Oct.	
	Francis Mukins	30 Mar. 1756	
	Henry Jodrell	31 do	
	John Maxwell, Senior	12 May	
	John Maxwell, Jun.	1 Sept.	
	Henry Hamilton	2 do.	
	Richard Nugent	21 Sept. 1757	4 Sept. 1745
	Isaac Aug D'Aripé	25 do.	
	Thomas Mitchell	26 do.	
	Andrew Cathcart	27 do.	
	Robert Ross	28 do.	
	Henry Howarth	29 do	
	William Prescott	30 do.	
	Francis Bolton	1 Oct.	
	Henry Nicholson	11 Jan. 1758	25 Dec. 1755
Ensign - -	James Leslie	27 Jan. 1757	
	William Irving	24 Sept.	5 Apr. 1756
	Rog Pomroy Gilbert	25 do.	
	William Skene	2 Oct.	
	John Lockhart	3 do.	
	Temple Walbanck	5 do.	
	Joseph Moneypenny	6 do.	
	AlexanderArbuthnot	11 Jan. 1758	3 Oct. 1757
Chaplain - -	George Lloyd	19 Feb 1756	
Adjutant - -	Francis Mukins	29 Aug. 1756	
Quarter Master	Edmond Worth	11 Jan. 1758	
Surgeon - -	Davis	13 Aug. 1756	

Agent. Mr.

I

Rank	Name.	Rank in the	
		Regiment.	Army
Colonel - -	Roger Handafyd	9 July 1730	Lt. Gen 29 Mar.43
Lieut. Colonel	John Laborde	2 Feb. 1757	
Major - -	Joseph Gabbett	2 Feb 1757	
Captain - -	John Harvey	11 July 1745	
	William Charters	31 Mar 1748	
	Henry Williamson	24 Jan 1752	
	William Agnew	15 Mar 1755	
	Dormer Harris	10 Dec.	
	Sir Tho Heron, Bt.	9 Apr. 1756	
	William Coxley	27 Aug. 1757	
Captain Lieut.	Thomas Lloyd	27 Apr 1756	
Lieutenant - -	Joseph Bland	24 Oct. 1747	
	Thomas Gaylard	15 Mar. 1755	
	John Plukenet	do.	
	William Davidson	10 Dec.	
	William Whyte	16 Feb. 1756	
	William Madden	do.	
	Bellingham. Chriftian	27 Apr.	12 May 1748
	Thomas Boyd	21 Sept.	
	Alexander Dickfon	11 Feb. 1758	
	Richard Leader	27 May	
Enfign - -	Fitzmorris Connor	27 Apr. 1756	
	James Alexander	do.	
	Charles Penefather	27 Nov.	
	Richard Vincent	do.	
	Charles Vero	do.	
	Charles Crawford	27 July 1757	
	Edward Courteney	3 Nov.	
	Stackpole Bailley	11 Feb. 1758	
	James Erfkine	27 May	
Chaplain - - -	Peter Peckard	10 Dec. 1755	
Adjutant - - -	William Madden	9 Apr. 1756	
Surgeon - - -	William Moore	23 Apr. 1757	

Agent, Mr. Defbrifay, Dublin.

Seven-

Rank.	Name.	Rank in the	
		Regiment	Army.
Colonel - -	John Forbes	25 Feb. 1757	
Lieut Colonel	Arthur Morris	21 Sept. 1756	
Major - -	John Darby	21 Sept. 15 6	
Captain - -	⎧Christopher Ruffell ⎪Edward Forfter ⎪Jocelyn White ⎨John Vaughan ⎪William Howard ⎪George Fulwood ⎩WmE. of Dundonald	1 June 1750 20 Aug. 1751 4 Sept 1754 21 Sept 1756 22 Nov. 2 Feb 1757 do	16 Oct 1748
Captain Lieut.	Paul Rycaut	2 Feb. 1757	
Lieutenant -	⎧Ch. Philpot Hughes ⎪Thomas Morris ⎪Philip Du Perron ⎪Edward Hope ⎨Charles Lyons ⎪Jonathan Rogers ⎪Capel St George ⎪William Watts ⎩Francis Tew George Swetteham	10 Dec. 1755 do. 27 Apr. 1756 21 Sept do. do 22 Nov. 2 Feb. 1757 do 27 Mar. 1758	
Enfign - -	⎧Rich. Mortgomery ⎪Willis Martin ⎪George Pafchall ⎪Michael Harrifon ⎨John Savage ⎪Henry Robinfon ⎪Samuel Williams ⎩Robert Williams John Chriftopher	21 Sept 1756 do. do 2 Feb 1757 do do do. 20 Mar 1758 21 do	
Chaplain - -	James Moore	16 Feb 1756	
Adjutant - -	Philip Du Perron	2 Feb 1758	
Quarter Mafter	Robert Williams	25 Feb 1757	
Surgeon - -	Jonathan Rogers	22 Jan 1755	

Agent, Mr. Rofs, Conduit ftreet.

Rank.	Name.	Rank in the Regiment.	Rank in the Army.
Colonel - -	John Folliott	22 Dec. 1747	Lt. Gen. 18 Jan. 58
Lieut. Colonel	Bigoe Armstrong	25 Nov. 1752	
Major - - -	Sir Rob. Hamilton, Bt. 14 Dec. 1755		
Captain - -	John Andrew Bigon	12 Oct. 1755	
	John Roberts	29 do.	
	Robert Batt	28 June 1756	
	Gustavus Moore	2 Feb. 1757	
	Henry St. John	12 Jan. 1758	
	Peter Wilbraham	26 May	
	Charles Edmonstone	27 do.	
Captain Lieut.	John Freake	27 May 1758	
Lieutenant -	Henry Folliott	24 Jan. 1752	31 Oct. 1745
	Isaac Hamilton	1 Oct. 1755	
	Charles Stuart	2 do.	
	Hugh Antrobus	3 do.	
	Richard Fauffet	31 Mar. 1756	
	John Stuart	18 May	
	Mathew Lane	23 June	
	Francis Wadman	20 Nov.	
	Blaney Brabazon	2 Feb. 1757	
	George Stamforth	27 May 1758	
Ensign - -	William Gauntlet	5 May 1756	
	Samuel Turner	17 do.	
	Lewis Wynne	18 do	
	Daniel Holroyd	28 June	
	Bigoe Armstrong	7 Oct.	
	Henry Whitehead	20 Nov.	
	Charles Durand	25 Feb. 1757	
	David Cooke	12 Jan. 1758	
	Arthur St. George	27 May	
Chaplain - -	Stanley Leathes	12 Mar. 1746	
Adjutant - -	Richard Fauffet	20 Dec 1755	
Surgeon - -	Samuel Scott	3 June 1752	

Agent, Mr. Desbrisay, Dublin.

Nineteenth

Rank	Name.	Rank in the Regiment.	Army.
Colonel - -	Ld. Geo. Beauclerck	15 Mar. 1747-8	Lt. Gen. 25 Jan. 58
Lieut. Colonel	Robert Douglas	10 Apr 1758	
Major - -	Charles Lumisden	23 Apr. 1758	
Captain - -	Robert Farmer	25 June 1744	6 Aug. 1740
	Alexander Moor	23 May 1746	
	William Rickson	21 Mar. 1752	23 Feb. 1747-8
	John Marriott	15 Oct. 1754	22 Feb. 1747-8
	John Wood	24 Apr. 1755	
	James Patterson	25 Aug. 1756	18 July 1755
	Thomas Pemberton	26 do	27 Apr. 1756
	Thomas Cuthbert	28 do.	
Captain Lieut.	George Borradale	16 Nov. 1757	Captain 19 Mar. 57
Lieutenant -	John Bird	24 Apr. 1755	
	John Scrymsour	2 Oct.	
	James Hebden	25 Dec.	
	James Lloyd	30 do.	
	Robert Harpur	13 Apr. 1756	
	William Bainbridge	14 do.	
	David Haldane	25 Aug.	31 Sept. 1754
	Duncombe Colchester	26 do.	3 Jan 1756
	John Pari	28 do.	27 Apr. 1756
	Alexander Gordon	29 do.	
	William Hatsell	30 Aug.	
	Robert Saville	5 Apr. 1757	
	Andrew Forbes	21 Sept.	
	John Majoribanks	22 do.	
	James Nugent	25 do.	
	John Evans	26 do	
	John Leslie	27 do.	
	William Gordon	28 do.	
Ensign - -	Henry Hutchinson	2 Sept. 1757	
	Robert Menzies	26 do	
	Archibald Bogle	27 do.	
	John M'Gill	28 do.	
	Dugal Stuart	1 Oct.	
	Thomas Wilson	3 do.	
	Henry Wastell	10 Feb 1758	
	John Stuart	5 June	
Chaplain - -	George Burvill	7 June 1751	
Adjutant - -	John Bird	14 Apr. 1756	
Quarter Master	William Bainbridge	20 Dec. 1755	
Surgeon - -	William Hamilton	25 Oct. 1748	

Agent, Mr. Adair, Pall-mall,

Twentieth

Rank.	Name.	Rank in the	
		Regiment.	Army.
Colonel - -	William Kingsley	22 May 1756	M. Gen. 20 Jan. 58
Lieut. Colonel	John Beckwith	21 Apr. 1758	
Major - - -	John Maxwell	8 May 1758	
Captain - -	Charles Grey	31 May 1755	21 Mar. 1755
	T. Worsop Lawrence	18 Oct	
	Joseph Frearson	28 do.	
	John Parr	4 Jan. 1756	
	Archibald Patoun	26 Aug.	Major 4 Jan 1758
	Walter Stewart	27 do.	27 Apr. 1756
	Alexander Tennant	29 do.	
Captain Lieut.	David Parry	9 Mar. 1757	
Lieutenant - -	Edmund Bradshaw	1 Oct 1755	
	John Thompson	3 do.	
	Edward Brown	26 Dec.	
	Thomas Charlton	27 do.	
	George Norbury	25 Aug. 1756	24 Dec. 1755
	George St. George	26 do.	27 Apr. 1756
	Henry Conyngham	27 do.	27 Apr. 1756
	Luke Nugent	28 do.	
	George Denshire	30 do.	
	Thomas Pringle	31 do.	
	William Walcott	1 Sept.	
	John Sponge	2 do.	
	James Clarke	3 do.	
	William Nugent	7 do.	
	Winthey Boswell	9 Mar. 1757	
	Francis Weyme	26 Sept.	
	John Brewer	27 do.	
	Thomas Thompson	29 do.	
Ensign - -	William Dent	3 Sept 1756	
	William Renton	24 Sept. 1757	
	John Craufurd	25 do.	
	Bolton Power	26 do.	
	Thomas Dawson	27 do.	
	John Stenhouse	28 do.	
	Nevin Irwin	30 do.	
	Charles Bourke	23 May 1758	
Chaplain - -	William Agar	17 Apr. 1755	
Adjutant - -	Thomas Charlton	26 Feb. 1756	
Quarter Master	James Clarke	27 June 1748	
Surgeon - -	George Fred. Boyd	5 May 1746	

Agent, Mr. Calcraft, Channel-Row, Westminster.

Twenty-

Rank.	Name.	Regiment	Army.
		Rank in the	
Colonel - -	Wm. E of Panmure	29 Apr. 1752	Lt. Gen 24 Jan. 58
Lieut. Colonel	Edward Maxwell	27 Apr 1758	
Major - -	Adam Levingſton	8 May 1758	
Captain - -	Robert Buchanan	13 Feb. 1750	1 June 1747
	Robert Gordon	12 Oct 1751	
	Hon. John Colvill	8 Aug. 1755	
	James Chiſholme	20 Dec. 1756	
	Charles Colvill	17 Sept. 1757	
	Meade Vaniewen	8 May 1758	
	Robert M'Gachan	do.	
Captain Lieut.	John Chiſholme	8 May 1758	
1ſt. Lieutenant	John Napier	7 Aug. 1749	
	Robert Bridges	30 Apr 1751	
	Duncan Campbell	16 Mar. 1754	
	David Hope	5 July 1755	
	Patrick Innes	27 Oct.	
	Charles Buckworth	28 Dec.	
	Patrick Campbell	2 Sept. 1756	
	John Gibſon	20 Dec.	
	Thomas Home	17 Sept. 1757	
	Joſeph Aikman	8 May 1758	
2d Lieutenant	Hugh Paterſon	27 Oct 1755	
	Neil Campbell	29 Dec.	
	James More	20 Sept 1756	
	Meydwell Maſon	10 Mar 1757	
	John Gordon	10 Feb 1758	
	John Wallace	1 Mar.	
	Peter Pruce Prowett	19 June	
	Joſeph Ramage	1 July	
	Henry Congalton	2 do.	
Chaplain - -	James Gordon	12 Jan. 1757	
Adjutant - -	Joſeph Aikman	21 Sept. 1757	
Quarter Maſter	James Chiſholme	26 Oct 1756	
Surgeon - -	Alexander Tough	10 Aug. 1745	

Agent, Mr. Wilſon, Craven-Street, the Strand.

		Rank in the	
Rank.	Name.	Regiment.	Army.
Colonel - -	Edward Whitmore	11 July 1757	
Lieut. Colonel	Andrew, Lord Rollo	25 Oct. 1756	
Major - - -	Robert Wrey	1758	
Captain - -	Samuel Zobell	5 Jan 1750-1	
	Thomas Johnston	22 Jan. 1755	
	John Campbell	16 Feb. 1756	
	Philip Townfhend	27 Apr.	
	Roger Shaak	21 Sept.	
	Christopher French	25 Oct.	
	Arthur Ormfby	1758	
Captain Lieut.	John Campbell	1758	
Lieutenant - -	Piers Butler	16 Feb. 1755	
	Hon. John Rollo	9 Apr 1756	
	Stephen Papon	27 do.	14 July 1749
	John Swift	do.	20 Jan. 1756
	Humphry Jones	21 Sept.	
	Robert Brifcoe	do.	
	Henry Brown	25 Oct.	
	William Hamilton	do	
	John Foxon	8 Mar. 1757	5 Jan. 1747-8
	Henry Alt	do.	21 Sept. 1754
	James Campbell	do.	4 July 1755
	John Williams	do.	1 Mar. 1756
	James St. Clair	do.	28 Nov.
	Henry Elwes	1 May	
	John Weft	2 do.	
	John Vickers	3 do.	
	John German	4 do.	
	Adam Williamfon	20 Nov.	
	Hill Hodgkinfon	22 do.	
Enfign - - -	John Stannus	9 Apr. 1756	
	Edward Brereton	27 do.	
	Edward Brabazon	do.	
	John Burke	21 Sept.	
	Agmondefham Vefey	do.	
	Cadwallader Wynne	do.	
	Burton Smith	25 Oct.	
	James Malcolm	8 May 1757	
	Thomas Townfhend	23 Nov.	
Chaplain - - -	Ifaiah Jones	28 May 1756	
Adjutant - - -	William Neale	21 Apr. 1758	
Quarter Mafter	Hon. John Rollo	26 Oct. 1756	
Surgeon - - -	Walter Henderfon	10 Dec. 1755	

Agent, Mr. Calcraft, Channel-Row, Weftminfter.

Rank.	Name.	Rank in the Regiment.	Rank in the Army.
Colonel - -	John Huſke	29 July 1743	L. Gen. 11 Aug 47
Lieut. Colonel	Ed. Sacheverel Pole	9 Jan. 1756	
Major - -	Thomas Marlay	7 Sept. 1756	
Captain - -	Charles Hemington	29 Oct. 1754	
	Paſton Gould	16 Oct 1755	
	Patrick Rainey	25 Dec	
	Paul Caſtleman	23 Mar. 1756	
	William Fowler	26 Aug.	27 Apr. 1756
	George Bingham	27 do.	27 Apr. 1756
	John Fox	28 do.	
Captain Lieut.	Richard Bolton	5 Apr. 1757	
1ſt Lieutenant	Benjamin Young	29 Oct 1754	
	Benjamin Bernard	2 Oct. 1755	
	William Inglis	3 Nov.	
	Cuthbert Shafto	26 Dec.	
	Charles Reynell	25 Aug 1756	27 Apr. 1756
	Joſeph Patterſon	26 do.	23 June 1756
	James Sutherland	27 do.	
	Harry Blunt	28 do.	
	Arthur Barber	1 Sept.	
	Philip Mercier	2 do.	
	Arthur Hawthorne	3 do	
	Grey Grove	25 Sept. 1757	
	George Orpin	26 do.	
	William Blakeney	27 do.	
	Robert Gibbings	28 do.	
	Thomas Grant	29 do.	
	Joſeph Ferguſon	30 do.	
	Frederick Mackenzie	3 Oct.	
2d Lieutenant	Charles Owen	9 Mar. 1757	
	Robert Maſon Lewis	5 Apr.	
	William Tyrwhitt	24 Sept.	
	James Creſwell	25 do.	
	Paul Ellers Scott	26 do.	
	William Wollery	27 do.	
	David Ferguſon	30 do.	
	George Pettener	1 Oct.	
Chaplain - -	James Aſhton	28 Sept. 1757	
Adjutant - -	Benjamin Bernard	23 Mar. 1756	
Quarter Maſter	Bailey	22 July 1758	
Surgeon - -	William Pearſon	15 July 1758	

Agent, Mr. Adair, Pall-mall

K

Rank.	Name.	Rank in the	
		Regiment	*Army.*
Colonel - -	Hon. Ed. Cornwallis	8 Feb. 1752	M Gen. 12 Feb. 57
Lieut. Colonel	William Rufane	27 Feb. 1750-1	
Major - -	William Prefton	26 Aug. 1756	
Captain - -	James Goring	11 June 1746	
	Jofeph Darby	22 Feb 1746-7	
	Henry Goddard	29 Apr. 1754	
	Robert Prefton	26 June	
	John Johnfton	25 Aug 1756	27 Apr. 1756
	John Berkenhout	26 do.	
	Richard Edwards	28 do.	
Captain Lieut.	John Hill	9 Mar. 1757	
Lieutenant -	Robert Carr	31 Mar 1756	
	John Henry Baftide	14 Apr.	
	Robert Sutton	18 May	
	Robert Johnfton	25 Aug.	2 Jan. 1756
	Ch. Kellond Courtney	26 do.	3 Jan. 1756
	Thomas Gladwin	27 do.	27 Apr. 1756
	Loftus Cathcart	28 do.	14 July 1756
	Hans Cleland	29 do.	
	Ralph Walfh	31 do.	
	George Thompfon	1 Sept.	
	Leonard Ord	2 do.	
	William Agnew	3 do.	
	John Rofs	4 do.	
	Charles Tairant	5 do.	
	Samuel Hughes	9 Mar. 1757	
	William Skinner	21 Sept.	
	Patrick Don	22 do.	
	Courtland Schuyler	do.	
Enfign - -	William Hunter	25 Sept. 1757	
	James Verchild	26 do.	
	Goodin Dehany	27 do.	
	Patrick Agnew	28 do.	
	Peter Margaret	30 do.	
	Andrew Jamarfon	2 Oct.	
	Arthur Albert	3 do.	
	Thomas Bell	4 do.	
Chaplain - -	Benjamin Span	19 Feb. 1754	
Adjutant - -	Samuel Hughes	20 Dec. 1756	
Quarter Mafter	Robert Carr	11 Feb. 1756	
Surgeon - -	Edward Gee	19 Sept. 1746	

Agent, Mr. Calcraft, Channel-Row, Weftminfter.

Twenty-

Rank	Name.	Rank in the	
		Regiment.	Army.
Colonel - -	William, Earl Home	29 Apr. 1752	M. Gen. 13 Mar 55
Lieut. Colonel	George Scott	22 Mar 1757	
Major - -	Thomas Goodricke	22 Mar. 1757	
Captain - -	David Home	4 July 1749	Lt. Col. 7 May 58
	Archibald Douglas	20 June 1753	
	Francis Gore	22 Jan. 1755	
	Robert Watson	5 July	
	George Roberts	21 June 1756	
	Archibald Don	22 Mar. 1757	
Captain Lieut.	Alexander Gordon	22 Mar. 1757	
Lieutenant -	Alexander Campbell	28 Aug. 1753	
	Adam Hay	22 Jan. 1755	
	John Lindsay	5 July	
	Henry Sterrop	3 Oct.	
	William Cashell	21 June 1756	
	Edmund Robinson	13 Aug.	
	Hon. John Napier	29 do.	
	Thomas Johnston	1 Sept.	
	Thomas Wilson	2 do.	
	Charles Home	22 Mar. 1757	
	Mathew Henderson	25 Sept.	
	John Wynne	26 do.	
	James Flint	27 do.	
	Ch. W. Le Geyte	28 do.	
	Richard Edgar	29 do.	
	Andrew Home	30 do.	
	David Wedderburne	1 Oct.	
	Lewis Vaflette	20 Dec.	
Ensign - - -	John Daniel	22 Mar. 1757	
	Samuel Pintard	24 Sept.	
	George Symmers	25 do.	
	Thomas Edgar	26 do.	
	Alexander Wade	3 Oct.	
	Wetwang March	4 do.	
	William Price	5 do.	
	John Gunning	20 Dec.	
Chaplain - -	Hon. Alex Home	31 May 1755	
Adjutant - ·	Henry Sterrop	17 Mar. 1746	
Quarter Master	John Wynne	25 Mar. 1758	
Surgeon - -	Augustine Chambers	5 May 1756	

Agent Mr. Calcraft. Channel-Row, Westminster

Twenty-

Rank.	Name.	Rank in the	
		Regiment.	Army.
Colonel - -	Philip Anftruther	31 Mar. 1720	Lt. Gl. 31 May 45
Lieut. Colonel	George Moncrieff	18 Dec. 1755	
Major - -	David Erfkine	22 Dec. 1755	
Captain - -	Charles Anftruther	23 Oct. 1745	
	Robert Prefton	15 Feb. 1745-6	
	Sir Rob. Arnott, Bt.	23 May 1746	
	Philip Skene	19 June 1751	
	Charles Erfkine	16 Dec. 1752	
	Sir K. Mackenzie Bt.	8 Aug. 1755	
	Dudley Templer	22 Oct.	
Captain Lieut.	Nicholas Kellaway	27 Apr. 1756	
Lieutenant -	Thomas Rigg	23 May 1746	
	Charles Prefton	20 June 1753	
	Thomas Afh	do.	
	Patrick Rigg	8 Aug. 1755	
	Edward Duer	1 Oct.	
	William Delaplace	2 do.	
	William Dalrymple	3 do.	
	Francis Shanley	27 Apr. 1756	
	William Anftruther	12 Jan. 1757	
	John Strong	13 do.	
Enfign - -	John Rofcrow	16 Dec. 1752	
	John Vere	3 Oct. 1755	
	Robert Weddall	5 May 1756	
	William Keir	27 Aug.	
	John Craufurd	28 do.	
	Robert Herbert	8 Nov.	
	Thomas Griffiths	12 Jan. 1757	
	William Colquhoun	18 May	
	Richard Baugh	12 Jan. 1758	
Chaplain - -	John Prefton	23 Feb. 1741-2	
Adjutant - -	Edward Ford	13 Jan. 1757	
Surgeon - -	Hopkins	8 Dec. 1756	

Agent, Mr. Defbrifay, Dublin.

Rank.	Name.	Rank in the Regiment.	Rank in the Army.
Colonel - -	Wm Ld. Blakeney	27 June 1737	Lt. Gen. 11 Sept. 47
Lieut. Colonel	William Haviland	16 Dec. 1752	
Major - -	Eyre Maſſey	10 Dec 1755	
Captain - -	Archibald Gordon	14 Oct. 1742	9 June 1740
	Anthony Wheelock	29 May 1747	30 July 1745
	Oſborne Jephſon	15 Apr. 1749	13 Apr. 1741
	John Wrightſon	16 Dec. 1752	20 Apr. 1748
	James Holmes, Sen	10 Dec. 1755	
	James Holmes, Jun.	2 Feb. 1757	
	Philip Skene	do	
Captain Lieut.	Henry Pringle	2 Feb. 1757	
Lieutenant -	Thomas Achmuty	10 Mar 1753	4 Sept. 1745
	Hugh Frazer	4 Sept. 1754	
	John Blakeney	10 Dec. 1755	
	Boyle Roche	do.	
	Robert Blakeney	27 Apr. 1756	
	Henry Symcocks	do	24 Jan. 1756
	Fred John Belcher	do.	
	William Cooke	do.	22 Jan. 1756
	Nicholas Netterville	21 Sept.	
	William Cotton	2 Feb. 1757	
Enſign - -	Peter Daly	16 Feb 1756	
	John Forteſcue	27 Apr.	
	Oliver Shorne	do.	
	Thomas Saunders	do.	
	Studholm	22 Nov.	
	John Elliott	do.	
	Thomas Williams	2 Feb. 1757	
	William Moore	25 Dec.	
	Francis Creed	27 Mar. 1758	
Chaplain - -	Henry Brown	19 June 1758	
Adjutant - -	William Moore	21 Sept. 1756	
Quarter Maſter	John Blakeney	13 Feb. 1757	
Surgeon - -	George Eagle	4 Apr. 1745	

Agent, Mr. Calcraft, Channel-Row, Weſtminſter.

Twenty

Rank.	Name.	Rank in the Regiment.	Army.
Colonel - -	Philip Bragg	10 Oct. 1734	L. Gen. 10 Aug. 47
Lieut. Colonel	Hunt Walſh	2 Feb. 1757	
Major - - -	John Dalling	2 Feb. 1757	
Captain - -	Thomas Addiſon	24 June 1744	9 June 1740
	Thomas Littler	30 Apr. 1746	24 Oct. 1745
	Ralph Corry	2 May 1751	
	Thomas Spann	28 Aug. 1753	
	Arthur Brown	10 Dec. 1755	
	James Mitchelſon	9 Apr. 1756	
	Aclomb Milbank	8 Mar. 1757	
Captain Lieut.	Joſeph Capel	8 Mar. 1757	
Lieutenant -	John Farmer	2 May 1751	
	James Halls	3 June 1752	
	Jerome Noble	22 Jan. 1755	
	Charles Taſſells	do.	
	Charles Ruxton	16 Feb. 1756	
	Francis Brown	9 Apr.	
	John Aſhe	27 do.	
	William Cooper	do.	
	William Phibbs	22 Nov.	
	William Evans	8 Mar. 1757	
Enſign - -	John Jervois	10 Dec. 1755	
	Synge Tottenham	16 Feb. 1756	
	Martin Fitzgerald	9 Apr.	
	Richard Gilmer	27 do.	
	Bingham Bourke	do.	
	John Sheppard	22 Nov.	
	William Bacon	do.	
	Eſſex Edgworth	8 Mar. 1757	
	Wm. Henry Fairfax	22 Nov.	
Chaplain - -	Ralph Walſh	12 Mar. 1754	
Adjutant - -	Charles Taſſell	9 Apr. 1756	
Quarter Maſter	Jerome Noble	9 Mar. 1757	
Surgeon - -	William Hewett	9 Apr. 1756	

Agent, Mr. Calcraft, Channel-Row, Weſtminſter.

Rank.	Name.	Regiment.	Army.
Colonel - -	Hon. Geo. Bofcawen	4 Mar. 1752	M. Gen. 14 Jan. 58
Lieut. Colonel	Henry Richardfon	23 June 1756	
Major - -	Bartholomew Blake	10 Dec. 1755	
Captain - -	Maurice Carr	16 Dec. 1752	
	Maurice Wemys	4 Sept. 1754	
	Archbold Dickfon	22 Jan. 1755	
	Edward Stopford	9 Apr. 1756	
	John Corrance	27 do.	
	William Lufhington	8 Mar. 1757	
	John Melvill	12 Jan. 1758	
Captain Lieut.	Mathias Knowles	27 May 1758	
Lieutenant - -	James Wyndus	4 Sept. 1754	
	Samuel Barrett	16 Feb. 1756	
	Robert Lyttelton	do.	
	John Hallowes	do.	
	Thomas Prefton	9 Apr.	
	Samuel Cathrens	22 Nov.	
	Kenith Alex. Price	8 Mar. 1757	
	Edward Whiting	3 Nov.	22 Nov. 1756
	William Goodwin	11 Feb. 1758	
	Thomas Travers	27 May	
Enfign - -	Berkeley Weftropp	16 Feb. 1756	
	John Courtney	9 Apr.	
	Charles Burton	27 do	
	Charles Lucas	22 Nov.	
	Charles Nefb.tt	8 Mar. 1757	
	James Johnfton	do.	
	Archibald Campbell	22 June	
	Robert Harrifon	11 Feb. 1758	
	John Goddard	27 May	
Chaplain - - -	Jofeph Cowper	16 Dec. 1752	
Adjutant - - -	Samuel Barrett	9 Apr. 1756	
Surgeon - - -	John Robertfon	10 Dec. 1755	

Agent, Mr. Chaigneau, Dublin.

Thirtieth

Rank	Name.	Rank in the Regiment.	Army.
Colonel - -	John, E of Loudoun	1 Nov. 1749	L Gen 22 Jan. 58
Lieut. Colonel	Sir Wm Boothby, Bt.	19 Mar.1749-50	
Major - - -	James Ramfay	28 Apr 1758	
Captain - -	James Rich	19 Aug. 1751	17 May 1748
	Thomas Smyth	20 do.	
	Henry Rugge	20 June 1753	
	George Lewis	12 Mar. 1754	
	John Wright	8 Aug. 1755	
	Hayman Rooke	4 Oct.	
Captain Lieut.	Henry Loftus	28 Aug. 1756	
Lieutenant -	Thomas Price	20 Aug. 1751	
	James Moutray	do.	
	William Snell	12 Mar. 1754	
	John Auguftine Jeuers	8 Aug. 1755	
	Charles Chapman	1 Oct.	
	Peter Dumas	28 Aug. 1756	
	Simon Digby	30 do.	
	Hen. Norton Jeuers	1 Sept.	
	Joseph Fitzgerald	2 do.	
	Wm Profper Popple	22 Mar. 1757	
	Vincent Conyngham	21 Sept.	11 Sept. 1754
	Chriftoph. Maxwell	25 do.	
	Loftus Nunn	26 do	
	John Winter	27 do.	
	John Muller	29 do	
	Thomas Dundas	30 do.	
	James Williamfon	1 Oct.	
	John McLelan	25 Mar. 1758	
Enfign - - -	Thomas Lee Warner	22 Mar 1757	
	Charles Abbott	14 May	
	Walter Batwell	29 July	
	Charles Clarke	3 Oct	
	Woodford Rice	4 do	
	Edward Johnfon	5 do.	
	Hairy Rooke	6 do.	
	John Jones	25 Mar. 1758	
Chaplain - -	Edward Thomas	9 Aug. 1756	
Adjutant - -	Charles Chapman	8 Aug 1755	
Quarter Mafter	Peter Dumas	9 Dec	
Surgeon - -	John Wright	26 Oct. 1756	

Agent, Mr Calcraft, Channel-Row, Weftminfter.

Thirty-

Rank.	Name.	Regiment	Army.
			Rank in the
Colonel -	Henry Holmes	8 May 1740	M Gen. 2 Feb 56
Lieut. Colonel	Hamilton Lambert	28 June 1751	
Major -	James Vignoles	28 Aug. 1756	
Captain -	Peyton Meares	6 Feb. 1752	
	Thomas Troughear	29 May 1753	
	Edward Bromley	25 Mai 1755	
	Robert Barker	17 Oct.	
	Henry, Earl of Suffex	28 June 1756	5 Mar 1755
	Patrick M'Douall	25 Aug.	23 June 1756
	Francis Laye	27 do.	
	Thomas Dunbar	28 do.	
Captain Lieut.	Caleb Woods	25 Aug. 1756	
Lieutenant -	Thomas Varloe	8 Aug. 1755	
	William Hooker	4 Oct.	
	James Campbell	30 Mar. 1756	
	Thomas Hodgson	31 do.	
	Thomas Maule	26 July	
	John Bolton	25 Aug.	27 Apr 1756
	John Warren	26 do.	27 Apr. 1756
	James Bruce	27 do.	
	Francis Vignoles	28 do.	
	James Moore	29 do.	
	Wager Ruffel	30 do.	
	Gregor Drummonds	31 do.	
	Thomas Pembroke	1 Sept.	
	Edward Croſton	6 do.	
	Joſeph Farmer	7 do	
	Alexander Neſbitt	22 Apr. 1757	
	Henry Sampſon	25 Sept.	
	Lewis La Chapelle	27 do	
Enſign - -	Richard Vicaridge	2 Sept. 1757	
	Alexander Campbell	26 do.	
	John Dorcas	28 do.	
	Hugh Dickſon	29 do.	
	Vernon Noake	30 do	
	Nicholas Stuart	1 Oct.	
	James Shaw	2 do.	
	John Ferguſon	3 do.	
Chaplain -	George Lillington	10 Dec. 1751	
Adjutant -	William Hooker	7 Feb. 1745-6	
Quarter Maſter	Lewis La Chapelle	17 Oct 1744	
Surgeon -	James Chalmers	1 Apr. 1744	

Agent, Mr. Fiſher, Axe-Yard, Weſtminſter.

L

Rank.	Name.	Regiment.	Rank in the Army.
Colonel - -	Francis Leighton	1 Dec. 1747	M. Gen. 5 Feb. 57
Lieut. Colonel	William M'Dowall	26 June 1758	
Major - -	James Seton	26 June 1758	
Captain - -	Archibald M'Nab	8 May 1749	7 Dec. 1745
	John Meslin	28 June 1751	
	He ry Debary	27 Nov. 1752	29 Feb. 1747-8
	John Quinchant	4 Mar. 1756	28 Apr. 1749
	Hans Hamilton	25 Aug.	27 Apr. 1756
	Charles Rofs	28 do.	
	John Kelfey	26 June 1758	
Captain Lieut.	George Farquhar	13 Feb. 1757	
Lieutenant -	Robert Farquhar	27 Aug. 1753	
	Ifaac Barre	1 Oct. 1755	
	John Nugent	3 do.	
	Montgomery Agnew	25 Dec.	
	Humphrey Hopper	27 do.	
	Milo Bagot	25 Aug. 1756	27 Apr. 1756
	Anthony Pujolas	26 do.	27 Apr. 1756
	William Mackay	27 do.	
	William Rickman	28 do.	
	Lawrence Norcop	30 do.	
	Andrew Armftrong	31 do.	
	John Horfley	3 Sept.	
	Richard Stukeley	2 Sept. 1757	
	William Southwell	24 do.	
	William Shewen	25 do.	
	Lewis Ray	26 do.	
	George Barclay	27 do.	
	Burnet Minific	26 June 1758	
Enfign - -	George Swiney	2 Sept. 1757	
	John Atkinfon	24 do.	
	William Ogilvie	25 do.	
	Thomas Coxe	27 do.	
	Edmund Vero	28 do.	
	Henry Cordwell	29 do.	
	John Drake	30 do.	
	William Daffy Cane	26 June 1758	
Chaplain - -	David Tanqueray	10 Oct. 1744	
Adjutant - -	George Farquhar	5 May 1756	
Quarter Mafter	Humphrey Hopper	30 Dec. 1755	
Surgeon - -	Peter Mackenzie	24 Dec. 1741	

Agent, Mr. Richardfon, Downing-ftreet, Weftminfter.

Rank.	Name.	Rank in the	
		Regiment	Army
Colonel - -	Lord Charles Hay	20 Nov. 1753	M. Gl. 22 Feb 57
Lieut Colonel	Ld G Hen Lennox	8 May 1758	
Major - -	Peter Daulhat	1 Sept. 1756	
Captain - -	Davis Toplady	25 June 1747	
	Tho Edmonstoune	24 July 1749	
	Barclay Cope	29 Apr 1752	
	George Drummond	4 Sept 1753	
	Robert Rayner	13 Sept 1754	
	Chichester Wrey	25 Aug. 1756	27 April 1756
	Burton Bindon	26 do.	27 Apr 1756
	Dunze Collins	27 do.	
Captain Lieut.	John Gore	18 Jan. 1757	
Lieutenant -	Anthony Isaacson	1 Oct. 1755	
	Alexander Gordon	3 do.	
	Henry Cotton	4 do.	
	Henry Creed	26 Dec.	
	Richardson Rynd	26 Aug. 1756	27 Apr. 1756
	Thomas Farnaby	27 do.	27 Apr 1756
	John Cuthbert	28 do.	
	David Calder	30 do.	
	Stephen Corfield	1 Sept.	
	Charles Butter	18 Jan 1757	
	William Blomberg	5 Apr	
	Jeremiah Tinker	21 Sept.	10 Apr 1755
	Thomas Walker	23 do.	Capt. Lt 4 Jan 58
	Terence Prendergast	24 do.	
	Hon. Ja Ruthven	27 do.	
	Thomas Duke	28 do.	
	James Coxeter	29 do	
	John Roberts	1 Oct.	
Ensign - -	Walter Kennedy	2 Sept. 1756	
	James Stewart	3 do.	
	James Dawson	4 do	
	William Young	24 Sept. 1757	
	Humphry Clarke	25 do.	
	Sackville Turner	30 do	
	Toby Close	2 Oct.	
	Simondson	3 do	
Chaplain - -	William Short	20 Dec 1755	
Adjutant - -	Henry Creed	25 Aug 1756	
Quarter Master	Alexander Gordon	8 Dec. 1756	
Surgeon - -	John Barker	5 May 1756	

Agent, Mr. Calcraft, Channel-Row, Westminster.

L 2

| Rank. | Name. | Rank in the | |
		Regiment.	Army.
Colonel - -	Tho E. of Effingham	2 Dec. 1754	M. Gen. 15 Jan 5
Lieut. Colonel	John Reed	7 Jan. 1756	
Major - -	John Dundas	2 Feb. 1757	
Captain - -	Joseph Widdens	10 Jan. 1756	
	John White	24 Aug.	
	James Hamilton	25 do.	28 Feb. 1755
	William Stacey	26 do.	8 Mar. 1755
	Boardman Bromhead	27 do.	19 Dec. 1755
	Robert Wilkie	29 do.	
	James Hamilton	30 do.	
Captain Lieut.	Thomas Kennan	1 Mar. 1758	
Lieutenant -	William Ogle	26 Nov. 1755	
	John Lind	29 Dec.	
	George Thorne	23 Mar. 1756	
	Conway Blizard	24 Aug.	
	William Ingram	25 do.	
	Daniel Shaw	26 do.	
	Hugh Mackay	27 do.	
	John Wylie	28 do.	
	Francis Mowatt	29 do.	
	William Sandys	2 Sept.	
	Langton Denshire	2 Feb. 1757	
	Christopher Lambert	2 Sept.	
	George Sutherland	24 do.	
	John Hamilton	25 do.	
	Julines Hering	27 do.	
	John Henery	28 do.	
	Hunter Sedgwick	1 Oct.	
	John Morrison	22 July 1758	
Ensign - -	Tho Dunster Hamar	22 Apr. 1757	
	George Duke	2 Sept.	
	John Gwynne	24 do.	
	William Johnston	25 do.	
	Lancelot Hilton	26 do.	
	George Smith	27 do.	
	Robert Elliot	5 Oct.	
	James Barclay	22 July 1758	
Chaplain - -	John Morgan	22 Mar. 1757	
Adjutant - -	Julines Hering	29 July 1757	
Quarter Master	John Lind	25 Aug. 1756	
Surgeon - -	Edward Bromhead	18 June 1757	

Agent, Mr. Winter, Brewer-street.

		Rank in the	
Rank	*Name.*	*Regiment*	*Army.*
Colonel - - -	Charles Otway	26 July 1717	Lt. Gen. 28 May 45
Lieut. Colonel	Henry Fletcher	16 Feb. 1758	
Major - - - -	Roger Morris	do.	
Captain - - -	⎧ John Maunfell	5 Jan. 1750 1	
	Thomas Collins	12 Mar. 1754	24 July 1746
	George Fletcher	8 Apr. 1755	
	⎨ William Bellew	16 Feb 1756	
	Charles Ince	24 do.	
	John Ormfby	do.	20 Nov. 1747
	⎩ Luke Gardiner	24 Jan. 1758	
Captain Lieut. -	Richard Baillie	24 Jan 1758	
Lieutenant - - -	⎧ Maurice Herbert	24 Jan 1752	
	John De la Vallê	11 Dec.	
	Thomas Jetherill	12 Mar. 1754	
	Edward Cant	7 Apr. 1755	
	William Bamford	16 Feb 1756	
	Richard Allen	do.	
	Thomas Brown	do.	
	Charles Gore	24 do.	
	Gabriel Maturin	12 April	
	⎨ Theophilus Blakeney	13 do.	
	Wm. Widdrington	14 do.	
	William Hamilton	15 do.	
	John Cockburne	26 Nov.	
	James Field	29 do.	
	Thomas Fortye	8 Mar. 1757	25 Nov 1755
	Wm. Fred. Phillips	16 May	
	William Mason	24 Jan. 1758	
	Eubule Ormfby	do.	
	James Abercromby	26 Mar.	
	⎩ William Brown		
Enfign - -	⎧ Nicholas Weld	16 Feb. 1756	
	Thomas Armftrong	9 April	
	Wm Ann. Skinner	10 do.	
	⎨ Colin Campbell	11 do.	
	Charles Portis	1 Dec.	
	Warham Browne	24 Jan. 1758	
	Cornelius Lyfaght	do.	
	Saunders		
	⎩ French		
Chaplain - -	Edward Whitty	9 Feb. 1750	
Adjutant - -	James Cockburne	25 Mar. 1757	
Quarter Mafter	William Hamilton	24 Feb. 1757	
Surgeon - -	Thomas Wilkins	22 Mar 1747	

Agent, Mr. Calcraft, Channel-Row, Weftminfter.

Thirty

Rank.	Name.	Rank in the	
		Regiment.	Army
Colonel - -	Ld. Robert Manneis	23 Mai. 1750-1	M. Gen. 7 Feb. 56
Lieut Colonel	Thomas Wilkinfon	11 July 1757	28 Dec 1755
Major - -	Gervas Remington	18 Jan. 1757	
	John Fleming	28 June 1751	
	Charles Forbes	13 Sept. 1754	
	Dudley Ackland	1 Oct. 1755	
Captain - -	Andrew Nappei	26 do.	
	Staates Long Morris	31 May 1756	12 Feb 1755
	Charles Webb	25 Aug.	7 Mar. 1755
	Henry Vaughan	27 do.	
	George Sheyne	28 do.	
Captain Lieut.	Peregrine Furye	9 Mar 1757	
	William Robinfon	19 Feb. 1756	
	Charles Pepper	20 do.	
	Richard Humpton	18 May	
	Cradock Wells	26 Aug.	
	Thomas Fouleiton	28 do.	
	James Bairy	29 do.	
	John Wittwiong	30 do.	
	Trefor Windei	31 do.	
Lieutenant -	Ed. Trotter Bannerman	1 Sept.	
	Michael Hare	2 do.	
	Thomas Woodcock	2 do.	
	John Pigott	21 Sept. 1757	19 June 1755
	Geo Cornwallis Brown	22 do.	
	Walter Sloane	23 do	
	Edward Tyng	24 do.	
	Jofeph Moore	26 do.	
	George Vaughan	27 do.	
	Francis Chefter	28 do.	
	Bazil Alves	27 Aug. 1756	
	Henry Popple	28 do.	
	Chriftopher Willoa	4 Sept.	
Enfign - -	John Bairy	6 do.	
	John Fowell	7 do.	
	Edmund Stiachan	8 July 1757	14 Mai 1757
	Archibald Erfkine	24 Sept.	2d. Lt 11 Mai. 1757
	Eccles Nixon	3 June 1758	
Chaplain - -	John Pearfall	18 Apr. 1748	
Adjutant - -	William Robinfon	17 Dec. 1754	
Quarter Mafter	James Bairy	31 Mai. 1756	
Surgeon - -	James Sturiock	29 Apr. 1757	

Agent, Mr. Fuije, Pulterey-ftreet.

Rank.	Name.	Regiment.	Rank in the Army.
Colonel - -	Hon. James Stuart	27 Nov. 1752	Lt Gen. 20 Jan. 53
Lieut. Colonel	Ja. Adol. Dickenson Oughton	7 Aug. 1749	
Major - -	Robert Hall	1 May 1758	
Captain - -	Loftus Cliffe	6 Feb. 1750	
	St George Dolley	21 Oct. 1755	
	Robert Daly	25 do.	
	William Turner	do.	10 Nov. 1755
	Anthony Blunt	26 do.	
	Henry Græme	25 Aug. 1756	2 Mar. 1755
	Robert Parkhurst	26 do.	24 Mar. 1755
	Joshua, Visc. Allen	27 do.	
Captain Lieut.	Francis Hutchinson	25 Aug. 1756	
Lieutenant -	Christopher Green	8 Apr. 1755	
	Peter Barbut	1 Oct.	3 June 1748
	George Slorach	3 do.	
	Edward Ormsby	4 do.	
	William Murdoch	25 Aug. 1756	25 June 1747
	James Gage	26 do.	
	James Coussean	27 do.	
	Alexander Stewart	28 do.	
	Dacre Hamilton	29 do.	
	Samuel Bowers	30 do.	
	Hugh Debbieg	1 Sept.	Capt. Lt. 4 Jan. 58
	Robert Brome	8 do.	
	Wm Montgomery	25 Sept. 1757	
	Robert Johnston	26 do.	
	John Smith	27 do.	
	James Slack	28 do.	
	Charles Mathews	29 do.	
	George Hog	1 Oct.	
Enfign - -	Nicholas Green	8 Oct. 1755	
	Boyle Spencer	9 Mar. 1757	
	Robert Newall	24 Sept.	
	Bolyn Douglas	23 do.	
	James Elliot	25 do.	
	Arthur Gregory	2 Oct.	
	Francis Graham	5 do.	
	William Charteris	15 July 1758	
Chaplain - -	James Moore	18 June 1742	
Adjutant - -	Christopher Green	31 Jan. 1756	
Quarter Mafter -	Edward Ormsby	31 Jan. 1756	
Surgeon - -	Robert Inglis	24 Sept. 1757	

Agent, Mr. Band, Downing-ftreet, Weftminfter.

Thirty-

Rank.	Name.	Regiment.	Rank in the Army.
Colonel -	James Lockhart Roſs	26 May 1756	
Lieut. Colonel	Nehem. Donnellan	14 Apr 1758	
Major -	Robert Melvill	8 Jan. 1756	
Captain -	Alexander Fraſer	26 Nov. 1751	
	William Gordon	17 Mar 1752	3 Sept. 1745
	De la Court Walſh	26 Mar. 1753	
	George Lucas	27 do.	
	William Horne	13 Oct. 1755	
	Joſhua Barker	26 June 1758	
Captain Lieut.	William Adlam	26 June 1758	
Lieutenant -	Wilſon Anderſon	27 Mar. 1753	
	Alexander Stewart	30 Mar. 1754	
	William King	28 Jan. 1755	
	Thomas Stevens	5 July	
	Richard Blathwayte	13 Oct.	
	William Archbould	31 Mar 1756	
	Thomas Playſtow	8 Dec	
	John Clarke	28 Nov. 1757	30 Aug. 1756
	Robert Young	10 Feb. 1758	5 Sept. 1756
	David Munro	26 June	
Enſign - -	John Kinkead	13 Oct. 1755	
	Gilbert Hillock	14 Apr. 1756	26 Feb. 1756
	Thomas Purnell	9 Dec.	
	James Trotter	10 do	
	David Ferguſon	27 Jan 1757	
	David Dawe	18 June	
	William Croſbie	16 July	
	Barnaby Rock	5 June 1758	
	Ja. Hilder Gamble	26 do.	
Chaplain - -	Cecil Willis	20 Dec. 1755	
Adjutant - -	Wilſon Anderſon	27 Mar. 1753	
Quarter Maſter	David Munro	12 Jan. 1757	
Surgeon - -	Robert Nicholſon	26 July 1756	

Agent, Mr. Roſs, Conduit-ſtreet.

Thirty-

Rank.	Name.	Rank in the	
		Regiment.	Army.
Colonel - -	John Adlercron	14 Mar. 1752	
Lieut. Colonel	Samuel Bagshawe	15 Apr. 1749	
Major - - -	Francis Forde	13 Nov 1755	
Captain - -	David Hepburne	7 Aug. 1746	
	Thomas Townsend	15 Apr 1749	
	Archibald Grant	9 Feb. 1750-1	
	Henry Wray	14 Feb. 1754	
	Nicholas Weller	19 Oct.	
	Eyre Coote	18 June 1755	
	Edward Hunt	19 do.	
	Anthony Walsh	13 Nov.	
	James Campbell	22 Apr. 1757	
Captain Lieut.	Charles Gually	13 Nov. 1755	
Lieutenant -	William Reynolds	19 June 1751	1 Nov. 1745
	John Corneille	14 Feb. 1754	29 Oct. 1745
	Christopher Hewetson	do.	
	John Fortescue	do.	
	Mathew Pearson	do.	
	John Carnac	18 do	30 Nov. 1745
	James Bush	19 Oct.	
	Caleb Powell	21 Feb. 1755	
	James Lewis	27 do.	
	Dominick Dalton	30 Nov.	
Ensign - -	John Power	16 Dec 1752	
	Joseph Adnett	14 Feb 1754	
	Martin Yorke	19 Oct.	
	Robert Fenton	25 Jan. 1755	
	James Horsburgh	26 do.	
	Bartholomew Balfour	19 May	
	George Cartwright	19 June	
	John Bradbridge	0 Aug.	
	John Donnellan	13 Nov.	
	Elias Clarke	8 Aug. 1756	
Chaplain - -	Plunkett Pieson	24 Jun 1752	
Adjutant - -	Dominick Dalton	20 Dec. 1755	
Quarter Master	Edward Fellx		
Surgeon - -	William Kerkct	10 Mar. 1715	

Agent, Mr Calcraft, Channel-Row Westminster.

Fortieth.

Rank.	Name.	Rank in the Regiment.	Army.
Colonel - -	Pereg. Tho. Hopfon	4 Mar. 1752	M. Gen. 11 Feb. 57
Lieut. Colonel	John Handfield	18 Mar. 1758	
Major - -	Chriftopher Aldridge	18 Mar. 1758	
Captain - -	George St. Loe	24 Nov. 1749	13 Apr. 1746
	George Scott	28 June 1751	
	John Hamilton	27 Mar. 1753	
	Otho Hamilton	26 June 1754	
	Samuel Cottnam	15 Oct.	
	Samuel Mackay	20 Nov. 1755	
	Walter Rofs	18 Mar. 1758	
Captain Lieut.	John Adlam	18 Mar. 1758	
1ft Lieutenant	George Cottnam	5 Sept. 1746	
	Robert Patefhall	25 Feb. 1748-9	
	William Handfield	1 Sept. 1749	
	Freke Dilkes Hore	24 Apr. 1750	
	Phillips Newton	29 July 1751	
	Hibbert Newton	15 Oct. 1754	
	Francis Gildart	12 Feb. 1755	
	John Hall	26 June	
	Thomas Myddleton	27 do.	
	George Parker	28 do.	
	Samuel Bradftreet	29 do.	
	Thomas Walker	30 do.	
	John Handfield	1 July	
	Wm. Aug. Gordon	2 do.	
	Henry Schomberg.	3 do.	
	Samuel Cameron	4 do.	
	Robert Robertfon	22 Nov.	
	Chriftoph. Aldridge	26 do.	
	Mofes Lilly	18 Mar. 1758	
2d Lieutenant	John Hamilton	28 June 1755	
	John Rofs	29 do.	
	Arthur Ormfby	30 do.	
	Alexander Winniet	1 July	
	Francis Green	2 do.	
	John Archbold	3 do.	
	Richard Sharpe	26 Feb 1756	
	Robert Catherwood	2 Apr. 1757	
	George Baftide	22 Mar. 1758	
Chaplain - -	George Thomfon		
Adjutant - -	John Adlam	7 Feb. 1757	
Quarter Mafter	John Hamilton	26 Feb. 1755	
Surgeon - -	Wm. Catherwood	7 Feb. 1757	

Agent, Mr. Adair, Pall-mall.

Rank	Name.	Rank in the	
		Regiment.	Army
Colonel - -	John Parſons	4 Mar. 1752	
Lieut. Colonel	Thomas Weldon	12 Feb. 1751	
Major - -	Edward Strode	12 Feb. 1751	
Captain - -	Chiverton Hartopp	23 Apr. 1742	Major 4 Oct. 1745
	William Roberts	25 Apr. 1751	29 Nov. 1745
	Lancelot Baugh	22 July	18 Apr 1743
	Philip Delegall	19 June 1752	
	John Muſgrave	10 Feb. 1753	18 Jan. 1740-1
	Charles D'Avenant	13 Oct. 1755	
	Cha. HubertHerriott	8 Nov. 1756	
Captain Lieut.	Joſeph King	19 June 1758	
Lieutenant - -	Francis Jeniſon	25 Jan. 1740-1	
	Henry Barnard	23 July 1748	3 July 1708
	John Phillmore	30 July 1753	10 Dec. 1745
	Robert Supple	19 Feb 1754	9 Feb. 1750-1
	George Boſſugue	26 Feb. 1756	23 Feb. 1755
	James Ouchterlony	26 July	15 Mar. 1747-8
	Joſeph Richardſon	18 June 1757	20 June 1735
	John Catherwood	19 June 1758	25 June 1744
	John Hudſon	do.	25 June 1755
Enſign - -	William Standert	24 Jan. 1740-1	
	Thomas Alford	18 June 1742	
	John Channon	30 July 1745	
	Thomas Morice	23 Dec.	
	Edward Stopforth	20 Mar.1745-6	
	Mathew Hall	17 Nov 1746	
	William Raper	23 July 1748	
	Robert Shepard	26 Sept. 1754	Lieut. 4 Oct 1745
	Patrick Douglas	28 June 1756	13 Nov. 1755
	Herbert Gibſon	8 Nov.	
Chaplain - - -	John Heber	25 May 1730	
Adjutant - - -	William Raper	14 Oct. 1755	
Quarter Maſter -	James Silk	20 Apr. 1751	
Surgeon - - -	John Swann	19 Oct 1721	

Agent, Mr. Furve, Pultney-ſtreet.

Rank.	Name.	Regiment.	Army.
			Rank in the
Colonel - -	Lord John Murray	25 Apr. 1745	Lt. Gl. 21 Jan. 1758
Lieut. Colonel	Francis Grant	17 Dec. 1755	
Major - -	{ Duncan Campbell	17 Dec. 1755	
Captain - -	{ Gordon Graham	3 June 1752	7 Aug. 1747
	John Reid	do.	
	John M‘Neil	16 Dec.	
	Allan Campbell	15 Mar 1755	
	Thomas Græme	16 Feb. 1756	
	James Abercrombie	do.	
	John Campbell	9 Apr.	1 Oct 1747
	James Stewart	18 July 1757	
	James Murray	20 do.	
	Thomas Stirling	24 do.	
	Francis M‘Lean		
	Archibald Campbell		
	Alexander St Clair		
	William Murray		
	Robert Arbuthnot		
	Alexander Reid		
	John Stuart		
Captain Lieut.	John Campbell	16 Feb. 1756	
Lieutenant - -	{ William Grant	22 Nov. 1746	
	Robert Gray	7 Aug. 1747	
	John Campbell	16 May 1748	
	George Farquarson	29 Mar. 1750	
	Kenret Tolmé	29 Jan. 1756	
	James Grant	24 do.	
	John Graham	25 do.	
	Hugh M‘Pherson	26 do.	
	Alexander Turnbull	27 do.	
	Alexander Campbell	28 do.	
	Alexander M‘Intosh	29 do.	
	James Gray	30 do.	
	William Baillie	31 do.	
	John Sutherland	10 Apr.	
	John Small	11 do.	
	Archibald Campbell	5 May	
	James Campbell	14 Dec.	
	Archibald Lamont	15 May 1757	
	David Mills	19 July	
	Simon Blair	20 do.	
	David Barclay	25 do.	

Lieutenant

Lieutenant -	Archibald Campbell	28 July 1757
	Alexander Mackay	1 Aug.
	Robert Menzies	2 do.
	Duncan Campbell	
	Alexander M'Lean	
	George Grant	
	George Sinclair	
	Gordon Clunes	
	Adam Stuart	
	John Robertfon	
	John Murray	
	john Grant	
	James Fiafer	
	George Leflie	
	John Campbell	
	Alexander Stuart	
	Duncan Richardfon	
	Robert Robertfon	

Enfign	Patrick Balnevie	28 Jan 1756
	Patrick Stuart	29 do.
	Donald Campbell	5 May
	James Mackintofh	15 Dec
	John Smith	15 May 1757
	Peter Grant	16 do.
	Duncan Stewart	17 July
	George Rattrav	19 do.
	Alexand. Farquarfon	22 do.
	Archibald Campbell	
	Archibald Campbell	
	Alexander Grant	
	M'Intofh	
	Patrick Sinclair	
	James M'Duffie	
	Thomas Fletcher	
	Alexan. Donaldfon	
	William M'Lean	
	William Brown	

Chaplain - - -	James Stewart	20 Dec. 1757
Adjutant - - -	James Grant	26 June 1751
Quarter Mafter	John Graham	19 Feb. 1756
	Adam Stewart	5 Aug. 1758
Surgeon - - -	David Hepburn	26 June 1751
	Rob. Drummond	5 Aug. 1758

Agent, Mr.   Drummond, Whitehall.

Rank.	Name.	Rank in the Regiment.	Rank in the Army.
Colonel - -	James Kennedy	7 Feb. 1745-6	M. Gen. 28 Jan. 56
Lieut. Colonel	Demetrius James	2 Feb. 1757	
Major - -	Robert Elliot	2 Feb. 1757	
Captain - -	Boughey Skey	2 May 1751	
	John Carter	20 June 1753	
	Richard Maitland	4 Sept. 1754	
	Roger Spendlove	9 Apr. 1756	
	Alex. Montgomery	21 Sept.	17 Aug. 1747
	James Talbot	2 Feb. 1757	
	David Maitland	21 Mar. 1758	
Captain Lieut.	David Alleyne	21 Mar. 1758	
Lieutenant -	William Dunbar	20 June 1753	
	Christopher Knight	12 Mar. 1754	
	John Knox	4 Sept.	
	Henry Clements	10 Dec. 1755	
	Vernon Hawley	16 Mar. 1756	
	Toby Purcell	9 Apr.	
	Blundel Dalton	27 do.	
	Robert Shaw	21 Sept.	
	Robert Molesworth	2 Feb. 1757	
	William Spread	25 do.	
Ensign - -	Nicholas Lysaght	9 Apr. 1756	
	Walter Nugent	27 do.	
	Trevor Hall	21 Sept.	
	Lewis Jones	22 Nov.	
	Thomas Arthur	do.	
	Crank Maw	do.	
	John Hatfield	2 Feb. 1757	
	Mounsieur Mercer	25 do.	
	Francis Le Hunte	2 Mar.	22 Nov. 1756
Chaplain - -	John Bourne	3 Jan 1740-1	
Adjutant - -	Christopher Knight	8 Aug. 1757	
Quarter Master	David Wilson	9 Mar. 1757	
Surgeon - -	William Younge	20 Aug. 1751	

Agent, Mr. Wilson, Craven-Street, the Strand.

Rank	Name.	Rank in the Regiment	Army.
Colonel - -	James Abercrombie	13 Mar. 1756	M. Gen. 31 Jan. 56
Lieut. Colonel			
Major - -	William Eyres	7 Jan. 1756	
Captain - -	John Beckwith	2 Mar. 1750-1	11 June 1748
	Francis Halkett	2 May 1751	
	Thomas Falkner	5 Nov. 1755	
	Charles Lee	11 June 1756	
	George Bartman	25 Dec.	
	Hon. Wm. Hervey	26 do.	
	Richard Bailley	6 June 1757	
Captain Lieut.	William Dunbar	6 June 1757	
Lieutenant -	John Treby	10 Mar. 1753	8 Sept. 1748
	Andrew Simpfor	26 June 1755	
	Robert Lock	27 do.	
	William Williams	28 do.	
	Daniel Difnie	29 do.	
	Robert Drummond	2 July	
	George Cleik	3 do.	
	William Prefton	4 Nov.	
	Thomas Hobfon	5 do.	
	George Pennington	6 do.	
	Thomas Gamble	7 do.	
	Thomas Eyres	8 do.	
	James Allen	9 do.	
	Ely Dagworthy	15 do	
	Francis Greenfield	11 June 1756	
	John Elwes	25 Dec.	
	Roger Kellet	27 do.	
	John Duncan	25 Apr. 1757	
	Primrofe Kennedy	6 June	
	Andrew Watfon		
Enfign - - -	Turbot Francis	25 Apr. 1757	
	Andrew Brown	9 May	
	Achilles Prefton	14 do.	
	Stephen Drayton	6 June	
	William Fiafer	23 Mar. 1758	
	Lawrence Smith		
	Samuel Johnfon		
	Edward Crofton		
	Allan M'Leod		
Chaplain - -	Philip Hughes	4 Jan. 1752	
Adjutant - -	Daniel Difnie	20 Jan. 1753	
Quarter Mafter	Richard Duncan	31 Mar 1758	
Surgeon - -	Robert Mackinley	30 July 1750	

Agent Mr. Calcraft, Channel Row, Weftminfter.

Rank.	Name.	Regiment	Army.
		Rank in the	
Colonel - -	Hugh Warburton	2 June 1745	Lt. Gl. 29 Jan. 1758
Lieut. Colonel	Montagu Wilmot	8 Apr. 1755	
Major - -	Alexander Murray	1 Oct. 1755	
Captain - -	William Cottrell	30 Ju'y 1745	
	William Walters	12 June 1747	
	Patrick Sutherland	24 Feb. 49-50	25 Apr. 1747
	James Clarke	12 Mar. 1755	
	James Cunningham	1 Oct.	
	John Cosnan	2 do.	
	Ralph Hill	18 Mar. 1758	
Captain Lieut.	Thomas Vaughan	19 Mar. 1758	
Lieutenant -	John Mitchell	1 June 1750	
	Gilfrid Collingwood	5 Mar. 1750-1	27 Feb. 1747-8
	John Pinhorne	26 May 1752	
	Broderick Fienca	10 Feb. 1753	
	Henry Dagdale	25 Nov. 1754	
	Richard Stevens	12 Mar 1755	
	Winkworth Tonge	8 Apr.	
	Richard Bulkeley	25 June	
	William Needham	26 do.	
	Cha Hufbands Collins	27 do.	
	John Bevan	28 do.	
	Walter Crosbie	29 do.	
	John Bowen	30 do.	
	John Wright	1 July	
	Edward Lee	2 do.	
	William Hall	3 do.	
	Erasmus John Phlips	1 Oct.	
	Theophilus Yonge	20 Mar 1756	
	Thomas Ervin	8 Mar. 1757	
	Hugh Nevin	18 Mar. 1758	
Enfign - -	Robert Wilmott	20 June 1755	
	Charles Shirreff	2 July	
	George Bains	3 do.	
	Charles Chetwode	1 Oct.	
	James Ormsby	30 Nov. 1756	
	Hans Wallace	18 Apr. 1757	
	James Biothe	25 Mar. 1758	
	Thomas Rous	26 do.	
Chaplain - -	Robert Brereton	11 Jan. 1740-1	
Adjutant - -	Cha Hufbands Coll ns	20 Mar. 1756	
Quarter Mafter	Edward Lee	7 Oct 1756	
Surgeon - -	Richard Veal	30 Sept. 1750	

Agent, Mr. Calcraft, Channel-Row, Weftminfter.

For)

Rank.	Name.	Rank in the	
		Regiment.	Army.
Colonel -	Thomas Murray	23 June 1743	Lt. Gl. 19 Jan. 1758
Lieut. Colonel	Samuel Beaver	2 Feb 1757	
Major -	William Browning	2 Feb. 1757	
Captain -	William Forbes	11 Feb. 1748-9	
	George Needham	29 Nov. 1749	
	Edward Wynne	4 Sept. 1754	
	Francis Legge	16 Feb. 1756	
	James Marsh	2 Feb. 1757	
	James Maxwell	do	
	William Leaver	3 do	
Captain Lieut.	Thomas Osborne	2 Feb. 1757	
Lieutenant -	Thomas Spencer	13 Dec 1752	
	Paul Mangin	16 Feb 1756	
	Robert Jocelyn	27 Apr.	
	Edward Downes	21 Sept.	
	William Hatfield	do.	
	Charles Osborne	2 Feb. 1757	
	Jacob Laulhé	do.	
	William Gordon	do	
	Arthur Lloyd	do.	
	John Wynne	3 do.	
Ensign - -	Mathew Johnston	21 Sept 1756	
	George Rogers	do.	
	Richard Cox	do.	
	Robert Brown	22 Nov.	
	William Philpot	2 Feb. 1757	
	George Crofton	do.	
	Pierce Butler	do	
	Thomas Carbonell	do.	
	Ann Gordon	3 do.	
Chaplain - -	John Dechair	10 Dec. 1755	
Adjutant - -	Thomas Bowden	23 Apr 1757	
Quarter Master	Thomas Carbonell	25 Feb. 1757	
Surgeon - -	Jonathan Mallet	31 Aug 1757	

Agent, Mr Drummond, Whitehall

N

Rank.	Name.	Rank in the Regiment.	Army
Colonel - - -	Peregrine Lascelles	13 Mar. 1742-3	Lt. Gen 16 Jan. 58
Lieut. Colonel	John Hale	19 Mar. 1758	
Major - - - -	John Huffey	19 Mar. 1758	
Captain - - -	William Spike	21 Apr. 1753	4 Aug. 1749
	Nicholas Cox	2 July	
	Samuel Gardner	27 Dec.	18 Sept. 1745
	John Spaal	24 Nov. 1755	
	John Mercer	10 Dec. 1756	
	Peter D'Arcy	11 Jan. 1758	
	Thomas Smelt	20 Mar	
Captain Lieut. -	Alexander Johnstone	20 Mar. 1758	
Lieutenant - -	Mathew Pattinson	12 Aug. 1750	4 July 1746
	Edward Malone	2 July 1753	
	Arthur Price	26 June 1754	
	Thomas Archbold	22 June 1755	
	Henry Goddard	23 do.	
	Wm. Nevill Wolseley	24 do.	
	William Sherriff	25 do.	
	Mathew Forster	26 do.	
	Henry Dobson	27 do.	
	Joseph Peach	28 do	
	Wm. Edw. Seymour	29 do.	
	Thomas Mercier	1 July	
	John Elphinstone	2 do.	
	John Forster	4 do.	
	Charles Basset	24 Nov.	
	George Mountain	9 Dec. 1756	
	John Morris	10 do.	
	Henry Mair	20 Mar 1758	
	James Stephenson	21 do.	
	Henry Stratford	28 do.	
Ensign - -	Thomas Gibson	1 July 1755	
	Milborne West	28 Nov 1756	
	Garnet Ewer	5 Dec.	
	Nicholson	10 do.	
	Harry Henning	1 Aug. 1757	
	John Price Guinet	18 Mar 1758	
	Kenneth Matheson	23 do.	
	William Farquhar	24 do.	
Chaplain - -	Bruce	22 July 1758	
Adjutant - -	Wm. Ed. Seymour	2 July 1757	
Quarter Master	Henry Goddard	24 Apr. 1755	
Surgeon - -	John Waterhouse	23 July 1757	

Agent, Mr. Calcraft, Channel-Row, Westminster.

Rank.	Name.	Regiment	Am.
		Rank in the	
Colonel - -	Daniel Webb	11 Nov 1755	
Lieut. Colonel	Ralph Burton	15 Oct 1754	
Major - -	Robert Rofs	20 Mar 1758	
Captain - -	Gabriel Chriftie	13 Nov 1754	
	John French	11 Feb. 1756	
	Somerville M'Queen	6 June 1757	
	John Gordon	21 Nov	
	Sir Ja. Cockburn Bt.	22 Mar. 1758	
	William Edmonftone	23 do.	
	Barry St Leger	24 do.	
Captain Lieut.	Theodore Barbut	21 Nov 1757	
Lieutenant -	Stephen Watehoufe	13 Nov 1754	
	John Hawthorn	25 June 1755	
	John Cope	27 do.	
	Jofhua Percival	1 July	
	Vere Royce	2 do.	
	John Dunbar	3 do.	
	James Montrefor	4 do.	
	Mat. Lefl.e	4 Nov.	
	James Cowart	6 do.	
	Allan M'Mullin	7 do.	
	Thomas Webb	9 do.	
	Richard Crow	10 do.	
	Robert Sterling	11 do.	
	Henry Moore	11 Feb. 1756	
	Thomas Hopkins	6 June 1757	
	John Lees	do	
	John Crofton	25 Jan 1758	
	Charles Davers	28 Mar.	
	John Hedges	29 do.	
Enfign - -	John Edmonftone	5 May 1757	
	Alexander Dowal	12 do.	
	Robert Frafer	17 do.	
	Godfrey Roe	6 June	
	Hen. La vs Lutterell	21 Nov.	
	Charles Humble	18 Dec.	
	Thomas Grove	25 Jan 1758	
	John Clarke	19 Mar.	
	Armftrong		
Chaplain - -	Michael Houdin	29 Apr. 1757	
Adjutant - -	John Hawthorn	6 Apr. 1758	
Quarter Mafter	Thomas Webb	29 Oct 1754	
Surgeon - -	Robert Murdock	28 Aug. 1755	

Agent, Mr. Calcraft, Channel-Row, Weftminfter.

Forty-

Rank.	Name.	Rank in the Regiment.	Army.
Colonel - -	George Walfh	22 Jan. 1754	
Lieut Colonel	Robert Spragge	29 May 1753	
Major - -	Park Pepper	29 May 1753	
Captain - -	William Newton	25 Dec. 1743	1 Nov. 1733
	Robert Hill	do.	2 Jan. 1738-9
	Robert Hodgfon	16 Aug. 1750	25 Dec. 1744
	James Crean	12 Jan. 1751	25 Dec. 1741
	James Trower	12 Aug. 1752	
	William Galbraith	27 Mar. 1753	
	Charles Shrimpton	18 June 1757	
Captain Lieut.	Iofhua Crump	18 June 1757	
Lieutenant -	John Verdon	15 Apr. 1748	
	Hugh Forfyth	23 July	
	Robert Myrie	1 Nov.	
	Hugh M'Kie	21 Dec.	
	Robert Hodgfon	28 Oct. 1749	
	Jeremiah Gardner	16 Jan. 1749-50	
	Sir Ja Campbell Bt.	31 Mar. 1750	
	James Lawrie	15 Aug	
	John Harris	10 Nov.	
	Charles Hinckes	7 June 1751	
	Bowater Vernon	7 Dec.	
	John Tutté	31 Jan. 1752	
	William Rofs	15 April	
	Thomas Dwarris	16 June	
	Walter Reddifh	12 Aug	
	Thomas Trelawney	9 Mar. 1753	
	Edward Pountney	10 do.	
	Luke Bourke	8 July	18 Aug. 1741
	John King	26 June 1754	
	Robert Brereton	5 July 1755	
	Charles Ofoorne	8 Aug.	
	Jofeph Spears	do.	
	Edw. William Pepper	26 Feb. 1756	
	Samuel Betts	2 Feb. 1757	
	Anthony Hixfon	18 June	
	Jones	29 July	
	William Cockburn	1 Dec.	
	Charles Stanhope	7 Mar. 1758	
	Peter Lewis Daulnis	5 June	
Chaplain - -	James Dyer	7 Oct. 1746	
Adjutant - -	John Smith	26 Oct. 1757	
Quarter Mafter	Sir Ja Campbell Bt	14 Oct. 1755	
Surgeon - -	Bowater Vernon	26 Feb. 1756	

Agent, Mr. Calcraft, Channel-Row, Weftminfter.

Fiftieth.

Rank.	Name.	Regiment.	Army.
		Rank in the	
Colonel	Studholme Hodgfon	30 May 1756	
Lieut. Colonel	John Mompeſſon	16 Dec. 1755	
Major	Lewis Thomas	2 May 1758	
Captain	Geo Auguſtus Barry	9 Oct. 1755	
	Thomas Calcraft	8 Nov.	
	George Mainwaring	27 Dec.	
	William Meulh	28 do.	
	Hugh Powell	30 do.	
	John Hey	do.	
	Sir Alex Hope, Bt	18 May 1756	
Captain Lieut.	John Woodward	27 Aug. 1756	
Lieutenant	Edward Pownall	3 Oct. 1755	
	Charles Lenn	4 do.	
	Alexand Hoiſburgh	20 Dec.	
	Samuel Pepper	2 Jan. 1756	
	Hugh Lowen	3 do.	
	Augrſtus Durnford	4 do.	
	James Denniſton	27 Aug	
	Robert Sutherland	25 Feb 1757	
	Henry Watſon	25 Sept.	
	Lodowick Cathcart	26 do.	
	Alexander Stuart	27 do.	
	William Bygrave	28 do.	
	Thomas Warburton	29 do	
	Pomeroy Gilbert	30 do	
	John Barry	1 Oct.	
	Lawrence Paget	19 Nov.	
	William Medows	20 do.	
	William Fleming	1 Mar. 1758	
Enfign	Henry Ogilvie	25 Sept. 1757	
	James Wood	1 Oct.	
	Edward Hamilton	2 do.	
	Baſkerville	3 do.	
	Edward Tiſdale	4 do.	
	Edward Hall	20 Nov.	
	George Denniſtoun	26 Jan. 1758	
	William Miller	1 Mar.	
Chaplain	John Black	15 Jan 1756	
Adjutant	Lawrence Paget	25 Feb. 1757	
Quarter Maſter	Alexander Stuart	27 Apr 1756	
Surgeon	Richard Turner	26 Jan 1756	

Agent, Mr. Adair, Pall-mall.

Rank	Name.	Rank in the	
		Regiment.	Aᵣmy.
Colonel - -	Thomas Brudenell	22 Apr. 1757	
Lieut. Colonel	Thomas Buck	20 Dec. 1755	
Major - - -	Noel Furye	16 Dec. 1755	
Captain - -	Hildebrand Oakes	3 Nov 1755	
	Rich. Montgomery	12 do.	
	John Blan	26 Dec.	
	Nehemiah Donellan	27 do.	
	William Martin	28 do.	
	William Baillie	29 do.	
	John Walker	30 do.	
Captain Lieut.	John Baldwin	26 Aug. 1756	
Lieutenant -	Andrew De la Cour	3 Oct. 1755	
	Lord Colvill	30 do.	
	Peter Cartwright	12 Nov.	
	Robert Biſſett	31 Dec.	
	Alexander Hamilton	1 Jan. 1756	
	Richard Brown	2 do.	
	William Roy	4 do.	
	Benjamin Dodd	26 Aug.	
	Robert Sinclair	25 Sept. 1757	
	John Widdows	26 do.	
	Nicholas Cotterell	27 do.	
	Richard Warburton	28 do.	
	Thomas Butterfield	29 do	
	Thomas Green	30 do.	
	Jonathan Hall	1 Oct.	
	Peter Gordon	25 Mar. 1758	
	.		
	.		
Enſign - -	William Culliford	2 Sept. 1757	
	Waine	2 Oct.	
	Samuel Knollis	3 do.	
	Robert Sherwood	4 do.	
	Brooke	5 do.	
	James Hogan	6 do	
	Joſeph Gill	26 Jan. 1758	
	Edward Fuller	19 June	
Chaplain - -	Thomas Maddock	19 Feb. 1756	
Adjutant - -	John Widdows	25 Dec. 1755	
Quarter Maſter	Peter Cartwright	12 Jan. 1757	
Surgeon - -	Francis Brough	26 Jan. 1756	

Agent, Mr. Guerin, Crown-Court, Weſtminſter.

		Rank in the	
Rank.	Name.	Regiment	Army.
Colonel - -	Edward Sandford	7 June 1758	
Lieut. Colonel	Alexander Mackay	21 Dec 1755	
Major - -	Hugh Morgan	18 Dec 1755	
Captain - -	Valentine Jones	13 Oct. 1755	
	Loftus Ant. Tottenham	30 do.	
	Henry Brownrigg	26 Dec	
	John Young	27 do.	
	Thomas Phillips	28 do.	
	John Travers	29 do.	
	Archibald Williams	30 do	
Captain Lieut.	Anthony Haslam	28 Aug 1756	
Lieutenant -	John Cooke	1 Jan 1756	
	Marmaduke Cramer	2 do	
	George Byng	3 do	
	Donald Grant	4 do	
	Nicholas Addison	21 do	
	William Borde	5 May	
	Newland Godfrey	18 do	
	Alexander McGwire	28 Aug	
	William Johnson	5 Apl 1757	
	Alexander Rose	7 May	
Ensign -	George Jefferson	3 Jan. 1756	
	Hon. Mark Napier	4 do.	
	Andrew Neilson	5 do.	
	William Dalrymple	21 do	
	John Dinsdale	1 May	
	Henry Powell	7 June	
	Leatherland	28 Aug.	
	John Bickerton	5 Apr 1757	
	Thomas Pilkington	7 May	
Chaplain - -	Richard Smith	13 Jan 1756	
Adjutant - -	William Dalrymple	21 May 1758	
Surgeon - -	Richard Hope	21 June 1756	

Agent, Mr. Cunning..., Dublin.

Rank.	Name.	Rank in the	
		Regiment.	Army.
Colonel - -	William Whitmore	21 Dec. 1755	M. Gen. 23 Jan. 58
Lieut. Colonel	William Arnot	31 Jan. 1758	
Major - -	John Lindesay	31 Jan. 1758	
Captain - -	George Sempill	19 Oct. 1755	
	Robert Lamb	31 do.	
	James Wakeman	5 Nov.	
	Thomas Benson	28 Dec.	
	Thomas Thompson	29 do.	
	James M'Farlane	30 do.	
	Geo. Oliph. Kinloch	31 Jan. 1758	
Captain Lieut.	John Slowe	27 Aug. 1756	
Lieutenant -	Robert Wright	29 Dec 1755	
	John Campbell	1 Jan. 1756	
	William Hughes	2 do.	
	Christopher Chambre	3 do.	
	John Donellan	4 do.	
	Cha. Lloyd Richards	18 May	
	George Massey	27 Aug.	
	Thomas Moore	25 Feb. 1757	
	Dugal Ewart	26 Oct.	
	John Wight	31 Jan. 1758	
Ensign - -	Lodovick Grant	2 Jan 1756	
	Westney Grove	5 do.	
	James Frognorton	20 Mar.	
	Peter Dondé	27 Aug.	
	Isaac Colnet	6 Aug. 1757	
	Grey Sparry	26 Oct.	
	Richard Davies	1 Dec.	
	George Digby	25 Mar. 1758	
	Arthur Harris	7 Apr	
Chaplain - -	George Watkins	31 Jan. 1756	
Adjutant - -	James Frognorton	21 do.	
Quarter Master	Westney Grove	6 Aug 1757	
Surgeon - -	William Adair	27 Jan. 1756	

Agent, Mr. Adair, Pall-Mall.

Rank.	Name.	Regiment	Army.
		Rank in the	
Colonel -	John Grey	5 Apr 1757	
Lieut. Colonel	Mark Kenton	23 Dec 1755	
Major -	Robert Walsh	10 May 1758	
Captain -	William Powell	3 Oct. 1755	10 Feb. 1753
	John Broughton	6 Nov	
	William Hamilton	26 Dec.	
	Geo Twisleton Rushleigh - do.		
	William Petere 23 co.		
	W am L do.		
	John Townsend 30 co.		
Captain Lieut.	John Debutts	27 Aug 1756	
Lieutenant -	Alexander Murray	2 Oct. 1755	
	John Price	3 do.	
	Edward Chester	do.	
	Alex Drummond	31 co.	
	Peter Beaver	1 Jan. 1756	
	William Skinner	2 do	
	Robert Bellenden	1 Feb.	
	Thomas Bird	5 May	
	Charles Philips	2? Aug.	
	George Maxwell	9 1757	
Ensign -	Henry Hamilton	29 Dec 1755	
	Robert Campbell	7 Jan. 1756	
	John Bowyer	7 do.	
	Andrew Peace	1 do	
	Robert Rainey	5 co	
	Hutton Dawson	7 June	
	Farq. Douglas	2? Aug.	
	Jona Baches	5 June 1758	
	Rowley Hill	5 Aug.	
Chaplain -	John Blair	15 Jan 1755	
Adjutant -	Ferq Douglas	31 do.	
Quarter Master	Alex Drummond	do.	
Surgeon -	John Scott	25 Jan 1756	

Agent, Mr White, Beerstreet

Rank.	Name	Rank in the Regiment.	Army.
Colonel - -	Geo. Aug Vilct. Howe	28 Sept. 1757	25 Feb. 1757
Lieut. Colonel	John Donaldson	25 Dec. 1755	
Major - -	Thomas Proby	24 Dec. 1755	
Captain - -	James Hargreaves	5 Oct. 1755	
	George Weft	7 Nov.	
	Withrington Morris	26 Dec.	
	Alexander Breden	27 do.	
	Alexander Duncan	28 do.	
	John Wilkins	30 do.	
	Alex Monypenny	22 Feb. 1757	29 Aug. 1756
Captain Lieut.	James Murray	29 Aug. 1756	
Lieutenant -	Thomas Baugh	26 Dec 1755	1 Oct. 1745
	Daniel Sullivan	28 do.	
	William Botteler	29 do.	
	James Minnett	31 do.	
	John Louthe	2 Jan. 1756	
	George Stuart	3 do.	
	William Soubiran	31 do.	
	Geo Le Hunt	14 Apr.	
	John Wharton	9 July	
	William Winepress	29 Aug.	
Enfign - -	Valentine Gardner	4 Nov. 1755	
	George Coventry	25 Dec.	
	Hugh Rofe	26 do.	
	William Downing	27 do.	
	Thomas Lloyd	3 Jan. 1756	
	John Luke	4 do.	
	John Gillan	5 do.	
	Hercules Ellis	29 Aug.	
	John de Berniere	22 Nov.	
Chaplain - -	Charles Paulett	15 Jan. 1756	
Adjutant - -	William Winepress	13 Mar 1756	
Quarter Mafter	French	18 June 1757	
Surgeon - -	Robert Darby	25 Feb. 1757	

Agent, Mr. Calcraft, Channel-Row, Weftminster.

Rank	Name.	Rank in the	
		Regiment.	Army
Colonel - -	LordCharlesManners	25 Dec 1755	
Lieut. Colonel	Peter Pair	26 Dec 1755	
Major - -	John Dorne	27 Dec. 1755	
Captain - -	James Stewart	1 Nov. 1755	
	William Skipton	26 Dec	
	John Heighington	27 do.	
	William Playfowe	28 do	
	John Deaken	29 do	
	John Ingram	5 Aug 1758	
Captain Lieut.	Wilfon Maffall	5 Aug. 1758	
Lieutenant -	James Pearn	3 Oct 1755	
	John Forfter	12 Nov	
	Thomas Harrifon	31 Dec.	
	John Archer	1 Jan. 1756	Capt. 4 Jan. 1758
	Edward Erle	2 do	
	David Dundas	3 do	
	John White	4 Mar.	
	St John Pierce Lacy	20 do	
	John Breteton	23 Aug.	
	Peter Parr	24 Sept. 1757	
	Edward Jenkins	25 do	
	Archibald Wright	26 do.	
	John Woorford	27 do.	
	Joseph Bodey	28 do.	
	John Hardy	29 do.	
	Thomas Langfon	1 Oct	
	George Kelk	25 Mar 1758	
	Wm RichardWillen	5 Aug.	
Enfign - -	William Lamplow	24 Sept 1757	
	Armftrong	25 do	
	John Sutherland	2 Oct	
	Thomas Stuart	3 do	
	Mackenzie	4 do.	
	George Garret	5 do.	
	Archibald Dunbar	19 June 1758	
Chaplain - -	John Helfred	31 Jan 1756	
Adjutant - -	John Hardy	do	
Quarter Mafter	William Lamplow	do.	
Surgeon - -	William Pitman	26 do	

Agent. Mr Turge, Fetterey-ftreet

O 2

Rank.	Name.	Rank in the	
		Regiment.	Army.
Colonel	Sr. David Cunynghame, Bt.	22 Mar. 1757	
Lieut. Colonel	Thomas Townſhend	3 Aug. 1757	
Major	George Onſlow	3 Aug. 1757	
Captain	Joſeph Harriſon	7 Oct. 1755	
	John Clifford	26 Dec.	
	William Craigg	28 do.	
	Daniel Clements	29 do.	
	Patrick Preſton	30 do.	
	Capt Ad. Kempenfelt	9 Mar. 1757	
	Thomas Weldon	7 Mar. 1758	
Captain Lieut.	Edw. Darterquenave	28 Aug. 1756	
Lieutenant	George Holliday	27 Dec. 1755	25 Sept. 1749
	Thomas Bennett	28 do.	
	Daniel Connelle	31 do.	
	Michael Cuffe	2 Jan. 1756	
	Edward Shaw	4 do.	
	William Slee	19 Feb.	
	Rd. Hickman	17 May	
	William Mocie	18 do.	
	Hon. Henry Keppell	26 Aug.	
	John Nicholls	28 do.	
Enſign	Sr. Wm. More Bt.	1 Jan. 1756	
	Ralph Adderſon	5 May	
	John Hutchion	2 Sept.	
	Hugh Roſe	26 Oct. 1757	
	James Phipps	1 Dec.	
	Wm. Toy	11 Jan. 1758	
	Thomas Pemberton	2 do.	
	George Robertſon	6 May	
	John Townſhend	8 July	
Chaplain	John Tooſey	12 May 1756	
Adjutant	Edward Shaw	4 Jan. 1756	
Quarter Maſter	Daniel Connelle	21 Jan. 1756	
Surgeon	Robert Knox	5 Aug. 1758	

Agent, Mr. Band, Downing-ſtreet, Weſtminſter

Fifty-

Rank	Name.	Rank in the Regiment	Army.
Colonel - -	Robert Anstruther	28 Dec. 1755	
Lieut Colonel	Hon. William Howe	17 Dec. 1757	
Major - -	James Agnew	17 Dec 1757	
Captain - -	Charles Graydon	26 Dec. 1755	
	John Nuttall	do.	
	George Byrd	27 do.	
	James Dalrymple	28 do.	
	Robert Rutherfurd	29 do.	
	John Leland	30 do.	
	Edward Smith	26 Jan. 1758	
Captain Lieut.	Edward Crymble	26 Jan. 1758	
Lieutenant -	Harrington Bardin	27 Dec. 1755	5 July 1755
	Abel Warren	30 do.	
	Horace Hayes	2 Jan. 1756	
	Jacques Brightman	4 Feb	
	David M'Kempte	11 do	
	James Stuart	5 May	
	Roger Woolcombe	28 Aug.	
	William King	26 Jan. 1758	
	John Grant	28 do.	
	Daniel Davis	11 Feb.	
Ensign - -	John Warburton	2 Jan. 1756	
	Jemmon Colley	4 do.	
	James Anstruther	27 Aug.	
	William Orme	28 do.	
	Boyle Spence	12 Jan. 1758	
	Charles Broughton	26 do.	
	James Watts	28 do.	
	William Call	11 Feb	
	Nicholas Tottenham	do.	
Chaplain - -	Hort Walker	4 Feb 1756	
Adjutant - -	David M'Kempte	11 Feb. 1756	
Quarter Master	James Stuart	1 May 1758	
Surgeon - -	Alexander Vere	26 July 1755	

Agent, Mr. Dalloes, Pall-mall.

Fifty

Rank.	Name.	Rank in the Regiment	Army.
Colonel - -	Charles Montagu	30 Dec. 1755	
Lieut. Colonel	Wm. Augustus Pitt	30 Dec. 1755	
Major - -	Joseph Lewis Feyrac	5 Jan. 1756	
Captain - -	James Manwaring	20 Oct. 1755	
	James Pringle	27 do.	
	Robert Milward	4 Nov.	
	Peter Hennis	28 Dec.	
	Allan M'Donald	30 do.	
	Robert Skeen	14 Apr. 1756	
	Enoch Markham	27 May 1758	29 June 1756
Captain Lieut.	Henry Reddish	27 May 1758	
Lieutenant -	Mathew Clerk	2 Oct. 1755	
	Joseph Williams	30 Dec	
	Hen Eglington Connor	31 do.	
	John Cooke	1 Jan. 1756	
	Robert Evans	2 do.	
	William English	18 May	
	Albert Jones	29 Aug.	
	Charles Moore	8 Mar. 1757	
	William Cowley	31 Mar. 1758	
	James Figge	27 May	
Ensign - -	George Herbert	2 Jan. 1756	
	James Munson	3 do	
	Thomas Martin	4 do	
	William Hucheson	5 do	
	John Clarke	29 Aug.	
	Alexander English	8 Mar 1757	
	Walter Borlase	12 Jan. 1758	2d Lt. 18 Mar. 1757
	George Bell	31 Mar.	
	Cornelius Helden	27 May	
Chaplain -	James Miller	15 Jan. 1756	
Adjutant -	John Clarke	31 do	
Surgeon - -	John Mubn	26 Jan. 1756	

Agent, Mr. Desbrisay, Dublin.

Rank.	Name.	Regiment.	Rank in the Army.
Colonel in Chief	James Abercromby 27 Dec 1757		M Gen 31 Jan 56
Colonel Commandant	{ John Stanwix } James Prevost } Charles Lawrence { Robert Monckton	1 Jan 1756 4 do 28 Sept. 1757 20 Dec.	
Lieut. Colonel -	{ Henry Bouquet } Frederick Haldiman } Sir John St Clair, Bt { John Young	3 Jan 1756 4 do. 6 do. 26 Apr 1757	
Major -	{ James Robertson } John Rutherfurd } Augustine Prevost { John Tulliekens	26 Dec. 1755 6 Jan. 1756 9 do 26 Apr 1757	Lt Col. 8 July 58
Captain -	{ Thomas Oswald Roco'p Faich Frederick Porter D Munster Walter Rutherfurd Charles Grame Ralph Harding Jeremiah Stanton Gmeling Richard Mather Geo. Wetterstroom Harry Charteris Sterrer } Francis Lander John Innis Burnand Gavin Cochran Joseph Prince Marcus Prevost Alexander Harbord Abrah Bosomworth John Bradstreet Thomas Jocelyn James DeLancy Samuel Willyamos George Du Fez Stephen Gually { William Stuart	26 Dec 1755 27 do 28 do. 29 do. 30 do. 1 Jan 1756 2 do. 4 do 5 do 6 do 7 do. 8 do 10 do 11 do. 13 do. 14 do 15 do. 16 do. 17 do. 19 do 20 do. 8 Mar 1757 do. do. do. do. 21 May 25 do.	 5 Sept. 1745 25 June 1747 25 Nov. 1754

Captain

Captain Lieut.	{ Edward Comberbach	28 Dec **1755**
	Schloffer	12 May **1756**
	Sam Jan. Hollandt	21 May **1757**
	Charles Forbes	22 Mar. **1758**

Lieutenant —			
Robert Brigftock	1 Jan. **1756**	16 Feb. 1747-8
Peter Von Ingen	2 do.	
Alexander M'Bean	3 do.	17 May 1748
Donald Campbell	4 do.	
Le Noble	6 do.	
John Longfdon	7 do.	
Allan M'Lean	8 do.	
Baziel Dunbar	12 do.	
Lewis Ourry	14 do.	
James Allaz	17 do.	
William Baillie	19 do.	
Chaft Spiefmacher	21 do.	
Elias Meyer	23 do.	
Simeon Lcuyier	25 do.	
Charles Willington	26 do.	
Charles Gallot	27 do.	
Grandidier	29 do.	
James Campbell	30 do.	
George Fullerton	1 Feb.	
Alexander Campbell	3 do.	
Jofeph Ray	4 do.	
George Turnbull	5 do.	
Wm Abercromoy	6 do.	
David Ouchterlony	7 do.	
William Hazlewood	8 do.	
John Brown	9 do.	
Daniel M'Alpin	10 do.	
Donald Forbes	11 do.	
Harry Gordon	12 do.	Capt 4 Jan. 1758
Thomas Baffet	14 do.	
George Faich	15 do.	
George Etherington	16 do.	
Emanuel Heife	17 do.	
Rodolphus Bentinck	18 do.	
Jacob Muller	19 do.	
Bernard Ratzer	20 do.	
Brehm. Diftrich	21 do.	
Fred Von. Weiffenfels	22 do.	
Jof.Fred Wallet des Barres	22 do.	
Conrard Gugy	24 do.	
Defnoilles	26 do.	
L. F. Fufer	27 do.	Lieutenant

	A. T. F Winter	28 Feb 1756	
	Von Ingen	29 do	
	Maier	12 May	
	Thomas Lindsey	28 do.	
	John Evans	29 do.	
	Brereton Peynton	30 Nov.	
	James Allen	1 Dec.	
	Thomas Bartley	2 do	
	George M'Intosh	3 do	
	Thomas Campbell	4 do	
	Ralph Phillips	5 do.	
	Samuel Mackay	6 do.	
	Francis Mackay	7 do.	
	George Archbold	8 do.	
	James Monro	9 do.	
	William Ridge	10 do.	
	William Hay	11 do.	
	Alexander Shaw	12 do.	
	Thomas Meredith	13 do.	
	Coes	18 do.	
Lieutenant	Bentley Glazier	8 Mar. 1757	21 Dec. 1754
	John Billings	do.	
	John Rodolph Khan	do	
	Peter Peniet	do.	
	John Folson	5 May	
	James Colyer	6 do.	
	Scot Campbell Carve	7 do.	
	Walter Kerr	8 do.	
	Michael Davis	9 do.	
	William Potts	10 do.	
	William Jones	11 do.	
	John Bell	12 do.	
	William Ryder	1_ do.	
	Thomas Winter	25 do.	
	James Ralfe	do.	
	Charles De Wildunger	25 July	
	Townshend Guy	22 Mar 1758	
	Robert Campbell	23 do.	
	James Crofton		
	James Jefferies	25 do.	
	John Wilson	26 do.	
	Francis Hutchinson		

P

Ensign

	James Herring	22 Jan	1756
	Edward Jenkins	23 do.	
	John Nuterville	25 do.	
	Allen Grant	1 Feb.	
	Alexander Grant	2 do.	
	George Otter	3 do.	
	Alexander Stephens	27 Nov.	
	Archibald Blane	4 Dec.	
	Dod Campbell	6 do.	
	William Ramfay	7 do.	
	Alexander Bailie	9 do.	
	Simon Frazer	10 do.	
	Lauchlan Forbes	11 do.	
	Thomas Pinckney	12 do.	
	William Brown	13 do.	
	John Leckie	14 do.	
	Alexander Shaw	17 do	
	Isaac Motte	19 do.	
Enfign	Ranflaer Schuyler	8 Mar.	1757
	Peter De Witt	3 May	
	John Dow	4 do	
	Francis Gordon	7 do.	
	William M'Lure	11 Jul	
	Arthur St. Clair	13 do	
	Alexander M'Intofh	18 do.	
	Henry Feyton	25 do.	
	Charles Rbor	22 July	
	James Weldier	16 Jan	1758
	Andrew Rofs		
	John Bay		
	J. Charles St. Clair		
	Haldimand	28 Mar	1758
	George Demler	29 do.	
	John Jamet	30 do.	
	Richard Fahie	31 do.	
	Louis Victor DuPleffis	1 Apr.	
	John Hav	2 do	

Chaplain

Chaplain - - -	Thomas Gawton	25 Dec. 1755
	W Nicholfon Jackfon	4 Feb 1756
	John Ogilvie	1 Sept. 1756
	Michael Schlaetler	25 Mar. 1757

Adjutant - - -	James Allen	18 Aug. 1756
	Thomas Barnfley	do.
	James Herring	13 June 1757

Quarter Mafter	Donald Campbell	18 Aug 1756
	Jofeph Ray	do
	James Samuel Engel	24 Feb. 1757
	Donald Campbell	6 June

Surgeon - - -	John M'Kenzie	Feb 1756
	George Wirgman	do
	Stevenfon	do
	Arthur Nicholfon	25 Dec.

Rank.	Name.	Rank in the	
		Regiment.	Army
Colonel - -	Grenville Elliott	21 Apr. 1758	M Gen 21 Apr. 58
Lieut. Colonel	John Barlow	18 Apr. 1758	
Major - -	Chriſtophe. Teeſdale	3 May 1758	
Captain - -	James Paterſon	27 Aug. 1756	27 Apr 1756
	Malby Brabazon	31 do	
	William Bulkeley	1 Sept.	
	Anketel Singleton	2 do.	
	Rowe. Crowe	3 do.	
	John Barford	18 Jan. 1757	1 July 1747
	Thomas Hardcaſtle	9 Mar.	
Captain Lieut.	William Gunning	2 June 1758	
Lieutenant -	John Acklom	25 Feb. 1756	27 Apr. 1756
	Peter Maturin	26 Aug.	
	Daniel Gilchriſt	27 do.	
	Walter Peyton	4 Sept.	
	Sampſon Pearce	5 do.	
	Thomas Brown	6 do.	
	John Rowland	7 do.	
	John Foote	8 do.	
	G. Venab. Chetwode	28 Sept 1757	
	John Veaugh	30 do	
	William Wilſon	1 Oct.	
	Robert Beatſon	2 do.	
	John Read	3 do.	
	Frederick Blombe g	4 do.	
	Redmond Kelly	5 do.	
	Nicholas Doolan	6 do.	
	Alexander Leſhnan	7 do.	
	John Badger	8 do.	
Enſign - -	John Skinner	27 Sept. 1757	
	John Ker	1 Oct.	
	James Savage	3 do.	
	John Ireland	4 do.	
	Edward Crowe	5 do.	
	John Arbuthnot	6 do.	
	Jarvis Palmer	22 July 1758	
	Samuel Horner	5 Aug	
Chaplain - -	George Chaw	8 May 1758	
Adjutant - -	William Gunning	26 Oct. 1757	
Quarter Maſter	Samuel Gay	25 Aug 1756	
Surgeon - -	Peter Joniſton	21 Sept 1757	

Agent, Mr. Fiſher, Axe-Yard, Weſtminſter.

Sixty

Rank	Name.	Rank in the Regiment	Army.
Colonel - -	William Strode	21 Apr. 1758	21 Mar. 1756
Lieut Colonel	John Jennings	15 Apr 1758	
Major - - -	Joieph Higginfon	8 Sept 1756	
Captain - -	Richard Temple	25 Aug. 1756	
	James Dalmahoy	30 do.	
	Jemet Cowait	31 do.	
	James Straton	1 Sept.	
	Vifco. Wallingford	2 do.	
	Richard Sherlock	3 do	
	John Monckton	28 Nov. 1757	
Captain Lieut.	Richard Legge	23 May 1758	
Lieutenant -	James Poole	29 Aug 1756	
	John Hand	4 Sept.	
	Richard Robins	5 do.	
	Thomas Nafh	6 do.	
	Benjamin Hall	7 do.	
	Barnabas Atkinfon	8 do	
	Wm MooreCaulfield	27 Sep. 1757	
	John Piggott	28 do.	
	Henry Harnage	29 do.	
	Thomas Sheppard	30 do.	
	Francis Rowland	1 Oct.	
	Earle Hawker	2 do.	
	Alexander Frafer	3 do.	
	Robert Aberciombie	4 do.	
	Thomas Corry	5 o.	
	Alex La Douefpe	6 do.	
	Alex Montgomery	7 do.	
	Dennis Davy	8 do.	
Enfign - -	Thomas Maltby	30 Sept. 1757	
	Swaine	1 Oct.	
	William Leigh	2 do.	
	John Saxton	3 do.	
	B ell S.l	4 do.	
	William Sturrt	5 do.	
	Sam Hen. Morgan	6 do.	
	George Seneys	25 Mar. 1758	
Chaplain - -	John Smyth	5 June 1758	
Adjutant - -	Benjamin Hall	19 June 1758	
Quarter Mafter	James Poole	13 Feb. 1757	
Surgeon - -	Edward Hawkins	7 May 1758	

Agent, Mr. Fifher, Axe-Yard Weftminfter

Rank.	Name.	Rank in the	
		Regiment.	Army.
Colonel - -	David Watfon	21 Apr. 1758	23 May 1756
Lieut. Colonel	Peter Defbrifay	17 Apr. 1758	
Major - -	John Trollope	30 Apr. 1758	
Captain - -	Robert Clevland	26 Aug. 1756	27 Apr. 1756
	Joferh Fifh	28 do.	
	John Bromer	29 do.	
	Henry Rogers	30 do.	
	John Ellis	31 do.	
	Charles Hamilton	1 Sept.	
	Charles Gilman	2 do.	
Captain Lieut.	George Cognian	26 May 1758	
Lieutenant -	Harcourt Mafters	3 Oct. 1755	
	John Anfruther	28 Aug 1756	
	John Philips Adams	30 do.	
	William Headley	2 Sept.	
	Thomas Jeffe	3 do.	
	James Ward	4 do.	
	John Ralph	5 do.	
	George Highton	6 do.	
	Mark Richards	7 do.	
	Michael Downes	1 Oct 1757	
	William Dexter	2 de.	
	Gerard Alt	4 do.	
	William Read	5 do.	
	James Hart	6 do	
	James Wyat	7 do.	
	Richard Nefbit	8 do.	
	Chriftopher Wefton	1 Mar 1758	
	Francis Colman	5 June	5 Oct. 175-
Enfign - -	William Denholme	25 Sept. 1757	
	Marlborough Liyan	27 do.	
	John Spence	5 Oct.	
	John Williams	1 Mar. 1758	
	John Kinneer	25 do.	
	John Haflewood	26 do.	
	George Peirs	27 do	
	Keith	28 do.	
Chaplain - -	William Adair	1 July 1758	
Adjutant - -	William Heatley	25 Aug 1756	
Quarter Mafter	Harcourt Mafters	25 Aug 1756	
Surgeon - -	John Morgan	24 Sept. 1757	

Agent, Mr. Adair, Pall-Mall.

Rank.	Name.	Rank in the Regiment	Army.
Colonel - -	John Barrington	21 Apr. 1758	25 May 1756
Lieut. Colonel	Wollaston Pym	11 Apr. 1758	
Major - -	Thomas Ball	25 Apr. 1758	
Captain - -	Alexander Leslie	25 Aug. 1756	25 Mar. 1755
	John Sneyd	28 do.	
	Alexander Summer	29 do.	
	John Woollarstain	30 do.	
	David Dickson	31 do.	
	William Forde	1 Sept	
	Watson Powell	2 do.	
Captain Lieut.	Bernard Rice	25 May 1758	
Lieutenant -	Nicholas Tench	26 Aug. 1756	23 June 1756
	William Maxwell	27 do	
	Charles Townshend	1 Sept.	
	John Day	2 do.	
	William Morrison	3 do.	
	Andrew M'Taggart	4 do.	
	John Roberts	13 June 1757	
	Thomas Acklom	21 Sept.	11 May 1748
	Thomas Walker	30 do	
	Curtis Farran	1 Oct.	
	Peter Calder	3 do.	
	John Williams	4 do	
	Gerald More	5 do	
	George Bell	6 do.	
	Mitchell Andrews	7 do.	
	Bordes Grand	8 do.	
	Robert Kington	26 Jan. 1758	
	Robert Howes	do.	
Ensign - -	George Browne	28 Sept. 1757	
	William Lucan	2 Oct	
	William Tidswell	5 do	
	John Nolan	20 Jan. 1758	
	William Lyon	27 do	
	Robert Lofty	28 do	
	Charles Bell	27 Mar.	
	William Abington	30 do	
	Robert Bell	5 Aug	
Chaplain - -			
Adjutant - -	Charles Townshend	27 Aug 1756	
Quarter Master	John Roberts	25 Aug 1756	
Surgeon - -	William Webb	24 Sept 1757	

Agent, Mr. Fisher, Axe-Yard, Westminster.

		Rank in the	
Rank.	*Name.*	*Regiment.*	*Army.*
Colonel - -	Robert Armiger	21 Apr. 1758	28 May 1756
Lieut. Colonel	John Salt	16 Apr. 1758	
Major - -	John DelGarno	29 Apr 1758	
Captain - -	Thomas Hall	27 Aug. 1756	27 Apr. 1756
	Teavil Appleton	28 do.	
	Charles Thompson	29 do	
	Hayward Stephens	30 do.	
	William Jenkins	31 do.	
	Charles Goulston	1 Sept.	
	Lovegood Watson	2 do.	
Captain Lieut.	Charles Weft Roberts	1 June 1758	
1ft Lieutenant	Lawrence Banyers	2 Oct. 1755	
	Duncan Campbell	5 Sept. 1756	
	John Gunn	6 do.	
	James Stephenson	23 Sept. 1757	
	Thomas Farell	24 do.	
	James Lyon	do.	
	William Butler	do.	
	Thomas Phillips	25 do.	
	Gillot Commelin	26 do.	
	William Roberts	27 do.	
	Edward Elfineie	28 do.	
	Nevil Parker	29 do.	
	William Dudley	30 do.	
	James Donaldion	1 Oct.	
	Frederick Sparkes	2 do.	
	John Vannei	3 do.	
	Eimes Gwillim	28 Nov.	
	G. Jocelyn Robinson	26 Jan. 1758	2 Oct. 1757
Enfign - - - -	James Mac Kay	5 Apr 1757	
	John Fluerty	7 May	
	William Carter	13 do.	
	Robert Morfe	24 Sept	
	Anthony Tolver	5 Oct.	
	John Middleton	26 Jan 1758	
	John Breefe	7 Mar.	
	Benjamin Paul	25 do.	
Chaplain - -	John Arrow	23 May 1758	
Adjutant - -	Anthony Tolver	5 June 1758	
Quarter Mafter	Lawrence Panyer	25 Aug. 1756	
Surgeon - -	Robert Brace	24 Sept. 1757	

Agent, Mr. Calcraft, Channel-Row, Weftminfter.

Roll.	Name.	Rank in the	
		Regiment	Army
Colonel - -	Edward Sandford	21 Apr. 1758	
Lieut Colonel	Rowland Phillips	23 Apr. 1758	
Major - -	Charles Beauclerck	7 May 1758	
Captain - -	George Daniel	29 Aug 1756	
	Anthony Sharpe	30 do.	
	Thomas Crofbie	31 do.	
	James Newton	1 Sept.	
	John Gillan	2 do.	
	James Johnfton	3 do.	
	Richard Mercer	21 do.	
Captain Lieut.	William Murray	27 May 1758	
Lieutenant -	Robert Drew	27 Aug 1756	13 Jan 1756
	William St. Clair	31 do.	
	John Evans	1 Sept	
	Andrew Agnew	2 do.	
	Thomas Watfon	3 do.	
	John Hill	4 do.	
	James Coates	29 Sept. 1757	
	Henry Goddard	30 do.	
	Rd Widmore Et.	1 Oct.	
	William Harrifon	2 do.	
	Algernoon Warren	3 do.	
	George Danfey	4 do.	
	John Penfon	5 do.	
	Andrew Rofs	6 do.	
	George Reynolds	7 do.	
	John Macharg	8 do.	
	John Barcas	10 Feb. 1758	
	William Grierfon	5 June	
Enfign - -	William Gregory	3 Sept. 1756	
	William Hepburn	29 Sept. 1757	
	Francis Bindon	2 Oct.	
	David Scott	5 do	
	Ifaac Smith	6 do.	
	Jocelyn Shawford	7 Mar. 1758	
	Richard Ellis	25 do.	
	Marfhal Wright	26 do.	
Chaplain -	Philip Francis	23 May 1758	
Adjutant -	John Barcas	15 July 1758	
Quarter Mafter	William Murray	25 Aug. 1756	
Surgeon - -	James Douglas	24 Sept. 1757	

Agent, M.. Colcraft, Channel-Row, Weftminfter.

Rank.	Name.	Rank in the	
		Regiment.	Army.
Colonel - -	James Wolfe	21 Apr. 1758	21 Oct. 1757
Lieut. Colonel	Robert Robinson	26 Apr. 1758	
Major - - -	Alex. Mac Duval	9 May 1758	
Captain - -	Francis Gregor	25 Aug. 1756	
	Charles Vearton	30 do.	
	Ed. Goodenough	31 do.	
	William Delaune	1 Sept.	
	Paul Meyer	9 Mar. 1757	
	James Dunne	1 Dec.	5 Apr. 1757
Captain Lieut.	Thomas Osborn	3 June 1758	
Lieutenant - -	George Sherwin	28 Dec 1755	
	James Nesbit	4 Sept. 1756	
	William Pughe	5 do.	
	William Edwards	6 do.	
	Francis Raper	25 Sept. 1757	
	Frecheville Dykes	28 do.	
	Marmaduke Green	30 do.	
	John Gardner	1 Oct.	
	John Cane	2 do.	
	Richard Faulkner	3 do.	
	George Smith	4 do.	
	William Yorke	5 do.	
	Philip Hales	6 do.	
	Henry Nesbit	7 do.	
	Thomas Wilkinson	9 do.	
	Alexander Rose	10 do.	
	William Socket	26 Jan. 1758	
	John Matson	3 June	
Ensign - - -	Richard Pilkington	2 Oct. 1757	
	Despard Croasdale	3 do.	
	William Herdsman	4 do.	
	William Massey	5 do.	
	Thomas Barker	6 do.	
	Joseph Collings	25 Mar. 1758	
	Royston Barton	22 July	
Chaplain - - -	George Carleton	26 June 1758	
Adjutant - - -	James England	8 July 1758	
Quarter Master	James Kirkman	24 May 1758	
Surgeon - - -	Joseph Harris	24 Sept. 1757	
	Agent,		

Rank	Name.	Rank in the	
		Regiment	Army
Colonel - -	John Lambton	22 Apr 1758	
Lieut Colonel	William Adey	22 Apr 1758	
Major - -	William Napier	6 May 1758	
Captain - -	William Rowley	25 Aug. 1756	24 Dec. 1755
	William Dundas	29 do	
	Peter Hewit	30 do.	
	Richard Lloyd	31 do	
	Tritham Revell	1 Sept.	
	John Birquire	2 do.	
	Richard Ridley	3 do.	
Captain Lieut.	Samuel Leslie	29 May 1758	
Lieutenant -	Joseph Dacre	30 Aug. 1756	
	Thomas Jenkins	31 do	
	Lewis Below	4 Sept	
	Edward Evens	7 do.	
	John Hatsell	8 do	
	George Munro	25 Feb. 1757	
	John Hunt	2 Oct.	
	Philip Patranche	4 do	
	William Alderton	5 do	
	Patrick Wikie	6 do	
	Thomas Armstrong	7 do.	
	William Teudale	9 do.	
	Humphry Hopper	10 do	
	William Prewitt	16 Feb. 1758	13 Feb 1757
	Bealter Brereton	7 Mar.	
	Thomas Nicholson	8 do	
	Arthur Owen	22 July	
	Robert Stafford	do.	
2d Lieutenant	William Tindale	2 Oct. 1757	
	William Melville	3 do	
	John Upton	4 do.	
	Philip Ibie	5 do.	
	Charles Wm Estc	27 Jan. 1758	
Ensign -	James Charles	22 July	
	George Hastings	23 do	
Chaplain - -	Lewis Bordeaue	8 July 1758	
Adjutant - -	George Munro	22 Jul 1758	
Quarter Master	George Munro	25 Aug 1756	
Surgeon - -	Thomas Bristowe	5 Aug. 1758	

Agent, Mr. Colcraft, Channel-Row, Westminster.

Q 2

Sixty

Rank.	Name.	Rank in the	
		Regiment.	Army.
Colonel - -	Hon. Char. Colville	23 Apr. 1758	
Lieut. Colonel	John Browne	24 Apr. 1758	
Major - - -	Edward Martin	22 Apr. 1758	
Captain - -	Aaron Clayton	27 Aug. 1756	
	Benjamin Bromhead	29 do.	
	William Mompesson	30 do.	
	Peter Boileau	31 do.	
	G. Montagu Martin	2 Sept.	
	James Macrae	3 do.	
	Thomas Pooke	4 do.	
Captain Lieut.	Ralph Haughton	24 May 1758	
Lieutenant -	Thomas Blunt	30 Aug. 1756	
	Valentine Green	7 Sept.	
	Abraham Scott	8 do.	
	Philip Baggs	25 Sept. 1757	
	James Paterson	26 do.	
	John Bowes Benson	27 do.	
	John Jeffer	28 do.	
	Thomas Horton	29 do.	
	James Ashe	30 do.	
	John Moore Travers	1 Oct.	
	Edward Ridley	2 do.	
	John Bromhead	3 do.	
	Thomas Tydd	4 do.	
	John Tate	5 do.	
	Edmund Stafford	6 do.	
	Henry Calowell	7 do.	
	Joseph Lovell	26 Jan 1758	
	Thomas Goddard	do.	
Ensign - -	Thomas Jones	5 Oct. 1757	
	John Wall	6 do.	
	William Mehew	26 Jan 1758	
	William Jackson	27 do.	
	William Moore	28 do.	
	Charles Head	25 Mar.	
	Thomas Milner	26 do.	
Chaplain - -			
Adjutant - -			
Quarter Master	Ralph Haughton	25 Aug. 1756	
Surgeon - -	William Morrison	24 Sept. 1757	

Agent, Mr. Calcraft, Channel-Row, Westminster

Seventieth

Rank	Name	Rank in the Regiment.	Army.
Colonel	John Parflow	27 Apr 1758	
Lieut. Colonel	Charles Vignoles	13 Apr 1758	
Major	Robert Pigot	5 May 1758	
Captain	William Piers	26 Aug. 1756	27 Apr. 1756
	Daniel Hamilton	29 do.	
	Titchborne Crueber	30 do.	
	Hector Monro	31 do.	
	George Grant	1 Sept.	
	William Nesbit	2 do	
	Hon Spen Compton	2 Sept 1757	
Captain Lieut.	John Fowle	28 May 1758	
Lieutenant	Jean Crofton	1 Oct 1755	
	John Stevens	28 do. 1756	
	William Smith	3 do.	
	Robert Clements	4 do.	
	Mufferden Jonathan	6 Sept 1757	
	Edward Hicks	27 do.	
	John Dumergue	28 do.	
	Arthur Lysaght	29 do.	
	George Whichcot	30 do	
	Arthur Thompson	1 Oct.	
	Roger Bristow	2 do.	
	Charles Sutherland	3 do	
	Anthony Morgan	4 do	
	Henry Norman	5 do.	
	Usback Prendergaft	6 do.	
	William Tulloh	9 do.	
	James Cuffes	8 May 1758	
	Williamfon Leg Hooker	19 June	
Enfign	George Williamfon	25 Sept 1757	
	George Kinloch	4 Oct.	
	Robert Jephfon	5 do.	
	Charles Gordon	7 do.	
	Robert Onock	8 do	
	William Talbot	25 Mar. 1758	
	Robert Wilfon	26 do	
	John Rofenhagen	20 June	
Chaplain	Thomas Parflow	25 May 1758	
Adjutant	Wm. Leg. Hooker	25 Aug. 1757	
Quarter Mafter	George Williamfon	25 Aug. 1757	
Surgeon	Samuel Bright	24 Sept 1757	

Agent, Mr. Calcraft, Channel-Row, Weftminfter.

Rank.	Name.	Rank in the Regiment.	Army.
Colonel - -	William Petcot	29 Apr 1758	
Lieut. Colonel	William Tayler	12 Apr 1758	
Major - -	Robert Murray	24 Apr. 1758	
Captain - -	Patrick Blake	29 Aug 1756	
	Theodore Desvorles	30 do.	
	Charles Boisragon	31 do.	
	James Durnford	1 Sept.	
	Chi st.Creswell Paine	2 do.	
	James Stuart	13 Feb 1757	
	Viscount Fitzmaurice	5 June 1758	23 May 1758
Captain Lieut.	Rawlins Hillman	22 May 1758	
Lieutenant -	Peter Beasley	29 Aug. 1756	
	John Burchall	2 Sept.	
	Vivian Davenport	4 do.	
	Thomas Lea	5 do	
	Ruben John Green	13 Feb. 1757	
	Thomas Saunders	28 Sept.	
	James Adeane	29 do	
	John Brown	30 do	
	James Eustace	1 Oct.	
	John Scobie	2 do.	
	John Hamilton	3 do.	
	William Paradice	4 do.	
	Richard Meredith	5 do.	
	William Fitzgerald	6 do.	
	Lancelot Baugh	7 do.	
	James Hey	8 do	
	George Bunington	9 do.	
	Richard Whyte	20 Jan. 1758	
Ensign - -	Theophilus Debat	26 Sept. 1757	
	Richard Atherley	1 Oct	
	John Coulson	2 do.	
	William Rudge Horn	3 do.	
	Ed. Bullingbrooke	4 do.	
	George Crosbie	5 do.	
	Roderick Mackenzie	6 do.	
	Orange Stirling	20 Jan. 1758	
Chaplain - -	Charles Roberts	19 June 1758	
Adjutant - -	Rawlins Hillman	25 Aug. 1756	
Quarter Master	Ruben John Green	25 Aug 1756	
Surgeon - -	Hamilton Steele	24 Sept. 1757	

Agent, Mr Calcraft, Channel-Row, Westminster.

Rank.	Name.	Rank in the Regiment.	Army
Colonel - -	Ch. D. of Richmond	9 May 1758	
Lieut. Colonel	William Wilkinfon	19 Apr. 1758	
Major - -	Richard Piefcott	20 Dec. 1756	
Captain - -	William Morris	28 Aug 1756	
	John Pollock	30 do.	
	Nevifon Poole	31 do	
	Robert Owen	1 Sept.	
	Percival Purcell	2 do.	
	Robert Gordon	3 do.	
	Charles Hervey	18 Jan 1757	
Captain Lieut.	Charles Crofbie	30 May 1758	
Lieutenant -	Thomas Jones	2 Oct 1755	
	John Atkins	2 Sept. 1756	
	Francis Price	3 do.	
	Edward Evans	4 do.	
	William Wright	5 do.	
	Bold Rofs	6 do.	
	Jofeph Hulbert	7 do.	
	Jofeph Pounfett	25 Sept. 1757	
	James Gorry	26 do.	
	John Fitzpatrick	30 do.	
	Gordon Forbes	2 Oct.	
	Samuel Elwood	3 do	
	Thomas Getmin	4 do.	
	Robert Drummond	5 do.	
	Innis Denty	6 de.	
	James Lambom	8 do	
	John Bower	9 do	
	Hugh Lord	8 May 1758	
Enfign - -	John Jones	14 May 1757	
	Jacob Grofe	2 Sept	
	Cardonnel Toplady	29 do	
	Hugh Echlin	1 Oct.	
	James Morden	4 do.	
	J. Svineiton Dyer	5 do.	
	George Rigge	6 do.	
	James Wooller	19 June 1758	
Chaplain - -	John Buckrer	23 May 1758	
Adjutant - -	Thomas Jones	8 Dec 1755	
Quarter M. fer	Ambrofe Well	25 Aug 1755	
Surgeon - -	Robert Walth	24 Sept 1757	

Agent, M. Adyr, Pall-mal

Rank.	Name.	Regiment.	Rank in the Army.
Colonel - -	William Browne	30 Apr 1758	
Lieut Colonel	Hezekiah Fleming	27 Apr 1758	
Major - -	Thomas Shirley	26 Apr 1758	
Captain - -	John Barber	1 Sept 1756	
	Samuel Laley	2 do.	
	Joseph Otway	8 Dec.	
	Harry Innes	do.	
	Henry Delaval	2 Sept. 1757	
	Rob. Murray Keith	20 do.	
	Charles Long	1 Mar. 1758	
Captain Lieut.	John Poyer	4 June 1758	
Lieutenant -	James Ewart	3 Sept. 1756	
	William Robison	4 do.	
	Edward Scutt	5 do.	
	John Maxwell	6 do.	
	Thomas Cheeke	14 May 1757	
	Richard Bradshaw	26 Sept.	
	John Fenton	do.	
	William Fea	29 do.	
	Samuel Hughes	30 do.	
	Edmund Armstrong	2 Oct.	
	George Eeles	3 do.	
	John Irving	4 do.	
	John Angus	5 do.	
	Joseph Allen	6 do.	
	Lancelot Armstrong	7 do.	
	William Charles	20 Dec.	5 Mar. 1757
	John Curry	26 Jan. 1758	
	Ch. J. Johnson Fielding	1 Mar.	
Ensign - -	Robert Johnston	1 Oct. 1757	
	Robert Scott	2 do.	
	James Innes	4 do.	
	Philip Higginson	6 do.	
	William Murray	11 Jan. 1758	4 Oct. 1757
	Charles Higgins	26 do.	
	Thomas Armstead	1 Mar.	
	Thomas Vowe	25 do.	
Chaplain - -	Thomas Edwards	5 June 1758	
Adjutant - -	George Eeles	14 May 1757	
Quarter Master	John Maxwell	5 June 1758	
Surgeon - -	Alexander Hewatt	24 Sept 1757	

Agent, Mr. Guerin, Crown-Court, Westminster.

Rank.	Name.	Rank in the Regiment.	Army.
Colonel -	Hon. Sharington Talbot	25 Apr. 1758	
Lieut. Colonel	William Masters	25 Apr. 1758	
Major - -	Thomas Maule	4 May 1758	
Captain - -	William Wade	26 Aug. 1756	
	Ulysses Fitzmaurice	29 do.	
	Michael Fleming	30 do.	
	John Forbes	31 do.	
	John Wilkie	1 Sept.	
	Richard Taylor	9 Mar. 1757	
	Alexander Rigby	26 June 1758	
Captain Lieut.	Robert Din	26 June 1758	
Lieutenant -	David Skene	27 Aug. 1756	
	George Hutchinson	4 Sept.	
	Jacob Farrow	5 do.	
	William Dunn	6 do.	
	John Delgatty	7 do.	
	John Graham	8 do.	
	Thomas Budet	25 Sept. 1757	
	John Beaton	29 do.	
	Francis M'Millan	30 do.	
	David Douglas	1 Oct.	
	Deane Donovan	2 do.	
	Henry Calder	3 do.	
	Francis Knox	4 do.	
	Jon Smith	26 Jan 1758	
	Hamilton Gorges	do.	
	Hugh Mackry	5 June	27 Sept. 1757
	Benier Stubbs	19 do	
	Robert Tymperley	26 do.	1 Dec 1757
	Tho Holingsberry	27 do.	
	William Preston	28 do.	
Ensign - -	William Dalton	1 Oct. 1757	
	Rd Tho Witter	3 do.	
	Richard Bertie	4 do.	
	William Towell	5 do	
	Samuel Mathews	6 do	
	Charles M'Gee	26 Jan 1758	
	Richard Bullock	27 do.	
	Monsel	26 June	
	Ralph Ramsy	27 do.	
Chaplain - -			
Adjutant - -	David Skene	2 Aug 1757	
Quarter Master -	Thomas Budet	25 Sept 1757	
Surgeon -	Jon Calder	2 do. 1757	
.	Agent.		

R

Rank.	Name.	Rank in the Regiment	Army.
Colonel - - - -	Hon. John Bofcawen	1 May 1758	
Lieut. Colonel -	Jorden Wren	20 Apr. 1758	
Major - - - - -	James Stuart	27 Apr. 1758	
Captain - - - -	James Money	19 Feb. 1754	
	Maurice Cure	28 Aug. 1756	
	Thomas Buck	29 do.	
	Thomas Adams	30 do.	
	John Gmord Craven	31 do.	
	John Watton	1 Sept.	
	Francis Allefieu	2 do.	
Captain Lieut. -	James Skene	31 May 1758	
Lieutenant - - -	William Stephenson	14 July 1755	
	Thomas Gilbert	31 Aug 1756	
	Thomas Walker	2 Sept.	
	James Baillie	3 do.	
	Mathew Ottley	4 do.	
	John Collier	5 do.	
	Angus Mackay	6 do.	
	William Dundas	7 do.	
	Maum. Cophill Savage	30 Sept 1757	
	Walter Nugent	2 Oct.	
	James Montgomery	3 do	
	Hampden Evans	4 do.	
	Thomas Howe	5 do.	
	John Maxwell	6 do.	
	Charles Marfh	7 do.	
	William Colfton	8 do.	
	John Dale	9 do.	
	Patrick M'Kie	10 do.	
Enfign - - - -	John Neilfon	18 Jan. 1757	
	Edward Nickler	28 Sept.	
	John Chilvers	29 do.	
	John Gray	30 do.	
	William M'Carmick	1 Oct.	
	Alexander Scott	3 do.	
	William Campbell	4 do.	
	Bethuen Lindefay	6 do.	
Chaplain - - -	Charles Tarrant	23 May 1758	
Adjutant - - -	Thomas Gilbert	25 Aug. 1756	
Quarter Mafter -	William Stephenson	25 Aug. 1756	
Surgeon - - -	John Wifeman	26 Jan 1758	

Agent, Mr Poumies, Bolton-ftreet, Piccadilly.

Rank.	Name.	Rank in the	
		Regiment.	Army.
Colonel - -	George, Lord Forbes	22 Nov. 1756	31 Dec 1755
Lieut. Colonel	John Pomeroy	21 Nov. 1756	
Major - -	{ William Newton	22 Nov. 1756	
	{ Peter Chester	do.	
Captain - -	{ Chambre Hallowes	22 Nov. 1756	
	Robert Gresley	do	
	George Johnson	do.	
	James Bruce	do.	
	Aden Ley	do.	
	Hugh Bateman	do.	
	Thomas Bourne	do.	
	{ William Hawkins	2 Feb. 1757	
Captain Lieut.	David Hay	22 Nov. 1756	
Lieutenant -	{ Richard Bettesworth	22 Nov. 1756	
	James Macdonald	do.	
	Robert Jenny	do.	
	Mathew Bunbury	do.	
	Hardresse Lloyd	do	
	Richard Fleming	do.	
	Lewis Cromelin deBirnier	do.	
	John Cotterell	do.	
	Samuel Stead	do.	
	William Chartres	do.	
	William Peacock	do.	
	William Bury	do.	
	Charles Cowe	do.	
	Sheldon	do	
	{ Robert Fitzgerald	27 Aug. 1757	

2d Lieutenant

2d Lieutenant	Robertfon	22 Nov. 1756
	Knight	do
	John King Pierce	do.
	Lawe	do.
	William Blizzard	do.
	Mathew Burke	do.
	Gervas Hall	do.
	Edward O'Brien	do.
	Doyley Bromfield	do.
	Hugh Ferrar	27 Aug. 1757

Enfign	John Hayter	22 Nov. 1756
	George Bolton	do.
	Huber Burgh	do.
	James Burne	do.
	Henry Collis	do.
	Whitwell Butler	do.
	William Deuxell	do.
	Rowland Davis	do.
	John Reynell	27 July 1757
	John Atkinfon	27 Aug.

Chaplain	Lill	22 Nov. 1756
Adjutant	Robertfon	22 Nov. 1756
	John Atkinfon	4 Jan. 1757
Surgeon	Samuel Palmer	22 Nov. 1756

Agent, Mr. Defbrifay, Dublin.

Rank.	Name.	Regiment.	Army.
		Rank in the	
Lt.Col.Comm.Hon.Archib.Montgomery		4 Jan. 1757	
Major - - -	James Grant	5 Jan. 1757	
	Alexander Campbell	7 do.	
Captain - -	John Sinclair	4 Jan. 1757	
	Hugh M'Kenzie	6 do.	
	John Gordon	7 do.	
	Alex. M'Kenzie	8 do.	
	William M'Donald	14 do.	
	George Monro	15 do.	
	Roderick M'Kenzie	17 do.	
	Allan M'Lean	16 July	
	James Robertson	19 do.	
	Allan Cameron	22 do.	
Captain Lieut.	Alexander M'Intosh	4 Jan. 1757	
Lieutenant - -	Charles Farquarson	6 Jan. 1757	
	Alex. M'Kenzie	7 do.	
	Nicholas Sutherland	8 do.	
	Archibald Robertson	9 do.	
	Duncan Bayne	10 do.	
	James Duff	11 do.	
	Colin Campbell	13 do.	
	Alex M'Donal	17 do.	
	Joseph Grant	22 do.	
	Robert Grant	25 do.	
	Cosmo M'Martin	26 do.	
	John M'Nabb	29 do.	

Lieutenant -
{
Hugh Gordon   31 Jan. 1757
Donald M'Donald   1 Feb.
William M'Kenzie   3 do.
Roderick M'Kenzie   5 do.
Henry Monro   7 do.
Alex. M'Donald   9 do.
Donald Campbell   11 do.
Hugh Montgomery   21 July
James Maclean   27 do.
Alexander Campbell 29 do.
John Campbell   30 do.
James M'Pherfon   31 do.
Archibald M'Vicar   7 Jan. 1758
}

Enfign - - - -
{
Alexander Grant   4 Jan. 1757
William Hagart   6 do.
Lewis Houfton   8 do.
William M'Lean   10 do.
James Grant   12 do.
John M'Donald   14 do.
Ronald M'Kinnon   16 do.
George Monro   20 do.
Alex. M'Kenzie   22 April
John M'Laughlan   21 July
Archibald Craufurd 24 do.
James Bain   7 Jan. 1758
}

Chaplain - - Henry Monro 12 Jan. 1757
Adjutant - - Donald Stuart do.
Quarter Mafter Alex. Montgomery do.
Surgeon - - Allan Stewart do.

Agent, Mr. Calcraft, Channel-Row, Weftminfter.

Seventy-

Rank.	Name.	Regiment.	Army.
		Rank in the	
Lt. Col. Comm.	S.mon Frafer	5 Jan. 1757	
Major - - -	{ James Clephane	4 Jan. 1757	
	{ John Campbell	6 do.	
Captain - -	⎧ John M'Pherfon	5 Jan. 1757	
	⎪ John Campbell	9 do.	
	⎪ Charles Baillie	10 do.	
	⎪ Simon Frafer	11 do.	
	⎨ Don.ld M'Donald	12 do.	
	⎪ john M'D nell	13 do.	
	⎪ Thomas Frafer	16 do.	
	⎪ Sir Henry Seton	17 July	
	⎪ Alexander Cameron	21 do.	
	⎩ Thomas Rofs	23 do.	
Captain Lieut.	J. Craufurd Walkinfhaw	5 Jan 1757	
Lieutenant -	⎧ James Frafer	4 Jan. 1757	
	⎪ Simon Frafer	5 do.	
	⎪ Alexander M'Leed	11 do.	
	⎪ Hugh Cameron	12 do.	
	⎪ Ronald M'Donald	14 do.	
	⎪ John Cuthbert	18 do.	
	⎨ Charles M'Donell	19 do.	
	⎪ Rory M'Neill	20 do.	
	⎪ William M'Donell	21 do.	
	⎪ Archibald Campbell	23 do.	
	⎪ John Frafe	24 do.	
	⎪ Hector M'Donell	27 do.	
	⎩ Donald M'Bean	28 do	

Lieutenant

Lieutenant - - -	John Frafer	30 Jan. 1757
	Alexander M‘Donell	2 Feb.
	John Murray	6 do.
	Simon Frafer	8 do.
	Alexander Frafer	12 do
	Alexander Campbell	7 May
	John Douglas	18 June
	John Nairne	16 July
	Arthur Rofe	17 do.
	Alexander Frafer	22 do.
	John M‘Donell	23 do.
	Cofmo Gordon	24 do.
	David Baillie	26 do.

Enfign - -	Evan Cameron	5 Jan. 1757
	Allan Stuart	7 do.
	Simon Frafer	9 do.
	Archibald M‘Alifter	13 do.
	Alexander Frafer	15 do.
	John Chifholme	17 do.
	John Frafer	19 do.
	Simon Frafer	21 do.
	James Mackenzie	7 May
	Malcolm Frafer	18 July
	Donald M‘Neill	20 do.
	Harry Monio	23 do.

Chaplain - -	Robert M‘Pherfon	12 Jan. 1757
Adjutant - -	Hugh Frafer	do.
Quarter Mafter	James Frafer	do.
Surgeon - -	John M‘Lean	do.

Agent, Mr Rofs, Conduit-ftreet.

Rank	Name.	Rank in the	
		Regiment	Army.
Lt. Col. Comm.	William Draper	2 Nov 1757	
Major -	{ Cholmondeley Brereton 2 Nov 1757		
	{ Hon. George Monſon 18 do.		
Captain - -	{ John More	24 Nov. 1757	10 Mai 1747-8
	Robert Edward Fell	26 do.	5 July 1756
	William Wade	27 do.	3 Sept 1756
	Richard Vaughan	28 do.	9 Mar 1757
	Godfrey Knuttall	1 Dec.	2 Sept. 1756
	{ Francis Drake	2 do.	
Captain Lieut	John Stewart	24 Nov 1757	
Lieutenant -	{ Thomas Cheſhyre	24 Nov 1757	18 Sept. 1754
	John Murray	25 do	6 Oct 1756
	Jeremiah Sleigh	26 do.	9 do
	Henry La Douespe	27 do.	5 Apr 1757
	John Chiſholme	29 do.	7 May
	Franc. Dupont	30 do	8 July
	George Brown	1 Dec	29 do
	John Whaly	2 do.	1 Oct
	Alexander Strahan	3 do.	28 Sept 1743
	Thomas Morie	4 do.	
	John Chriſtian Eiſer	6 do	
	Thomas Brown	7 do.	
	Iſaac Robinſon	8 do.	
	John Murr	9 do.	
	Henry Upfield	10 do.	
	Tarran	11 do.	
	Thomas Sefton	26 Jan. 1758	
	{ Garth Brown	10 Feb.	
Enſign - - -	{ Samuel Hopkins	26 Nov 1757	7 May 1757
	William Reffell	27 do.	14 do
	William Winchelſea	28 do	18 June
	William Le Grand	29 do.	29 July
	William Popham	30 do.	do.
	James Rofton	26 Jan 1758	
	John Henry	10 Feb	
	{ .		
Chaplain - -	Caleb Colton	2 Nov 1757	
Adjutant - -	John Murr	19 Dec.	
Quarter Maſter	Thomas Cheſhyre	do.	
Surgeon - -	Samuel Smith	do	

Agent M.. Colcraft, Channel-Row, Weſtminſter.

S   Eightieth

Rank.	Name.	Regiment.	Rank in the Army
Colonel - -	Hon. Thomas Gage	5 May 1758	
Captain - -	James Dalyell	25 Dec. 1757	
	Henry Gladwin	26 do.	
	Quinton Kennedy	27 do.	
	Hugh Arnot	28 do.	
Captain Lieut.	John Parker	25 Dec. 1757	
Lieutenant -	Robert Bayard	26 Dec. 1757	
	Norman M'Cloed	27 do.	
	George Campbell	28 do.	
	Charles Wllyamoz	29 do.	
	Stephen Kemble	30 do.	
	Dunbar	31 do.	
	John Hall	1 Jan. 1758	
	Becher	2 do.	
Ensign - -	Droute	25 Dec. 1757	
	William Irwin	26 do	
	Frafer	27 do.	
	Ward	28 do.	
	Walter Paterfon	29 do.	

Surgeon - -

Agent, Mr. Calcraft. Channel-Row, Weftminfter.

Eighty-

		Rank in the	
Rank.	Name.	Regiment	Army
Colonel - -	Alex. Lord Lindores	7 Apr 1753	
Major - - -	{ Richard Bowles { William Brown	13 Oct 1755 3 Nov.	12 Mar 1742 12 May 1740
Captain - -	{ John Tucker William Marſhall John Noble Thomas Burton Wm Lord Newark Charles Terrott Samuel Criche	13 Oct. 1755 do. do do. do. do. 15 June 1756	13 June 1744 26 June 1744 1 May 1745 29 May 1745 20 Sept 1745 28 Feb. 1751 29 Nov. 1745
Captain Lieut.	{ Lambert Vannier { Samuel Buck Veal	13 Oct 1755 5 May 1756	1 Oct. 1755
Lieutenant -	{ Berry Irvin Thomas Hawkins Thomas Jeures James Chambers William Reade John Bigg Lewis Giant	13 Oct 1755 do do. do do 13 May 1757 12 Nov	5 Oct. 1747 29 Aug 1756
Enſign - -	{ Richard Cornmell Thomas Butler Thomas Pringle Peter Foubert Lachlan M'Intoſh John Templeton Samuel Roger Armſtronge Franke Mark Page	13 Oct. 1755 do do. do do. do 22 May 1757 14 May 15 June	Lieut 4 Oct. 1755 7 Oct 1745

Agent, M. Fonye, Pultney-ſtreet

Rank.	Name.	Rank in the Regiment.	Army.
Colonel - -	John Parker	8 Apr. 1758	
Major - - -	{ William Johnston { William Godfrey	13 Oct. 1755 8 May 1758	4 Oct. 1745 4 Mar. 1751
Captain - -	John Gugleman George Carr James Graham James Hamilton Thomas Smith Digby Berkéley Jonathan Forbes William Courtenay	12 Jan. 39-40 13 Oct. 1755 12 Nov. 13 do. 15 June 1756 8 Dec. 20 do. 20 Sept. 1757	 6 Oct. 1753 5 Jan. 1751 30 Oct. 1751 13 Oct. 1755 Major 11 June 1753 28 Aug. 1756
Captain Lieut.	Richard Francis	5 Apr. 1757	
Lieutenant -	Edmond Wiseman John Cliffe William Brown William Smith James Adear Adam Wood Mathew Bishop William Cleland	9 July 1739 13 Oct. 1755 do. 15 June 1756 do. 24 July 8 Nov. 12 Nov. 1757	 18 Apr. 1749 21 Nov. 1747 20 Sept. 1754
Ensign - - - -	Robert Heath Nevil Williamson Thomas Bickerton John Goldhawke James Moorhead Robert Lawson Donald Valentine Thomas Fenton Anthony Hoffman	9 Dec. 1745 17 Apr. 1755 13 Oct do 17 Mar. 1756 15 June do. 7 Oct. 14 May 1757	25 Jan. 1743-4 26 Dec. 1750 4 Oct. 1745

Agent, Mr. Furye, Pultney street.   Royal

Master General and Colonel, His Grace the Duke of Marlborough,
Colonel en Second Rt. Hon. Ld Geo Sackville, Lt. Gen. of the Ordnance.

Col. Com.	{ * William Belford } { Borgard Michelfen }	1l. 5s. p. Diem	8 Mar. 1750-1 4 Feb. 1757
Lt. Col.	{ George Williamfon } { Tho. Defaguliers }	1l. per Diem	3 Feb. 1757 4 Feb. 1757
Major	{ John Chalmers } { Thomas Flight. }	15s. per Diem	1 Mar. 1755 4 Feb. 1757

26 CAPTAINS 10s. per Diem
MASTER GENERAL.

Thomas Ord	1 Mar. 1745-6
James Pattifon	1 Aug 1747
Alexander Leith	1 Apr. 1749
Charles Brome	8 Mar 1750-1
John Godwin	1 Sept. 1751
Thomas James	1 Mar. 1755
Richard Maitland	do.
Samuel Cleveland	do
William Heflop	do.
Charles Farrington	29 Oct.
Jofeph Brome	1 Apr. 1756
Abraham Tovey	do.
William Huffey	12 May
William Phillips	do.
John North d	
Jacob Gregory	4 Feb. 1757
Samuel Strachey	do.
John Dovers	2 Apr.
William Martin	do,
John Innes	do.
Thomas Smith	do
Philip Webdal	4 Jan. 1758
Peter Innes	do
Leonard Pattifon	19 Ap..

Alexander Campbell	1 Apr. 1756
Forbes Macbean	do.
Francis James Buchanan	do.
George Charleton	12 May
David Hay	do.
James Stephens	do.
Jacob Tovey	do.
David Muckle	1 Dec.
John Yorke	4 Feb. 1757
George Anderfon	do.
Andrew Fergufon	2 Apr.
Robert Hind	do.
Benjamin Stehelen	do.
Duncan Drummond	do.
Charles Torriano	do.
James Butler	do.
Thomas Howdel	do.
John Molman	do.
Jofeph Winter	
Thomas Baker	4 Jan. 1758
George Lewis	do
David Rogers	do
David Day	do
Thomas Blomer	19 Apr.

26 CAPTAIN LIEUTS 6s. per D.em

Borgard Michelfen	29 Oct 1755
William Macleod	1 Sp. 1756

25 1ft LIEUTENANT, 5 per Diem

Charles Stranover	1 Apr. 1747
Edward Whitmore	1 Mar 1755
Gilfrid Williams	do.
Sir Charles Charlton	2, do
Jofeph Barr	do
Thomas Hand	29 No
	19 Ap.

* B... 1755

Jonathan Lewis	1 Dec. 1756	Thomas Heathcote	4 Jan 1758
John Carter	2 Apr. 1757	John Stewart	19 Apr.
Joseph Walton	do.	William Lee	do
Edward Foy	do.	Richard Chapman	1 May
Fleming Martin	do.		
Josiah Jeffreys	do		
Samuel Glegg	do.		
George Phoenix	do.		
Christopher Schalck	do		
Anthony Farrington	do		
Primrose Elphinston	do.	**76 LIEUT. FIRE-WORKERS, 3s. 8d.**	
William Gostling	8 June	George Groves	1 Mar. 1755
Thomas Rogers	4 Jan. 1758	John Chalmers	do.
Thomas Collins	do.	Daniel Sweet	do.
Alexander Johnson	do.	John Scott	do.
Henry Skynner	do.	Thomas Sanders	1 June
John Michelsen	do.	James Wood	1 Oct.
John Pomeroy	do.	Edward James	29 do.
John Williamson	19 Apr	Thomas Pitts	12 May 1756
John Wilson	do.	Benjamin Cock	9 July
		George Rochfort	do.
		Robert Patrickson	do.
		David Vans	
		Joshua Brereton	1 Aug.
		John Mean	1 Oct.
		George Elliot	1 Nov.
		Thomas Davis	1 Dec.
26 2d LIEUTENANTS, 4s per Diem.		William Congreve	4 Feb. 1757
Robert Hitzler	1 Aug 1756	John Benjamin	do.
Peter Trail	2 Apr. 1757	Charles Wood	do.
Ellis Walker	do.	J Simpson Spencer	do.
David Standish	do.	Frederick Chapman	do.
Thomas Jones	do	Edward Williams	do.
William Johnson	do.	Richard Hill	do.
Thomas Simpson	do.	Thomas Robinson	do.
Thomas Davis	do	James Macdonald	3 June
Joseph Eyre	do.	Alexander John Scott	do.
William Hill	do	John Sinclair	do.
Philip Martin	do	William Archer Huddleston	do.
William Borthwick	do.	David Scott	do.
Nathaniel Conner	do	Richard Harrington	do.
Agar Weetman	do	George Fade	do.
James Donnellan	4 Jan. 1758	Philby Lambert	do
William Harris	do	Walter Michelsen	do.
John Carden	do	Thomas Patterson	do.
Vaughan Lloyd	do	George Wright	do.
Edward Nethercote	do	James Sowerby	do
Robert Rogers	do.	William Godwin	do
Ingleby Moore	do.	John Lemoine	do.
			Robert

Robert Fenwick	8 June 1757	John Davidson	8 Feb. 1758
Thomas Johnson	do.	John Smith	do.
Sir George Wheate, Bart.	do.	Samuel Tovey	do.
George Stamper	do.	Archibald Mitchell	do.
John Robinson	do	David Price	19 Apr.
Richard Campbell	do	Charles Mason	do.
James Lewis Warren	do.	William Tiffin	do.
John Thiel	do.	John Dampier	do.
Henry Evans	do.	Edward Davis	do.
Francis Downman	do	Daniel Tyrdale	do.
Thomas Hofmer	do	Nathaniel Lindesley	do.
Thomas Deane Pearce	do	Joseph Gaston	1 May
Thomas Young	do	Thomas Lewis	do.
Isaac White	1 Oct.	Benjamin Solly	do.
Lachlan Shaw	8 Feb 1758	William Lillot	19 do.
Stephen Adve	do.	.	
Alexander Maclelan	do.		
Alexander Jordan	do.		
John Enetzeke	do		
Daniel Goil	do		
William Adams	do		
James Fermer	do		

STAFF-OFFICERS.

Chaplain, Montagu Barton,		24 Dec. 1753	0	6	8
Adjutant { Forbes Macbean		1 Apr 1756	0	5	0
Duncan Drummond		4 Feb. 1757	0	5	0
Q. Master { John Pomeroy		1 June 1756	0	6	0
Thomas Baker		4 Feb. 1757	0	6	0
Bridge Master George Anderson		4 Feb. 1757	0	5	0
Surgeon———James Irwin		15 Dec. 1749	0	4	0
Surgeons Mates { William Hobson		1 Mar. 1755	0	2	6
Edward Taylor		6 May 1758	0	2	6

Agent, Mr. Cockburn, King-street, Golden-square.

Artillery Company of Ireland, all dated 1 April, 1756

Major, Henry Brownrig	15s.	Wm. Brady, J Retch, R. Graham
Captain, James Stratton	10	5 Serjeants, 2s. 6d. 1 Corp 1s 10d
1st } Lt { George Skipton	5	106 Bombardiers, 1s 8d
2d } { William Gray	4	34 Gunners, 1s. 4d. 102 Matross 1s.
3 Lt. Fire-workers, 3s 8d. each.		2 Drummers, 1s each
		Engineers

Rank.	Name.	Corps.	Army.
Chief as Colonel	William Skinner	14 May 1757	
Ch. Director in America as Col.	John Henry Baftide	4 Jan. 1758	
Director as Lieut. Colonel.	James Montresor	4 Jan. 1758	
Sub. Director as Major.	Wm. Cuninghame	4 Jan. 1758	Lt. Col 7 May 57
	Archibald Patoun	do.	
	Patrick Mackellar	do.	
Engineer in Ordinary as Captain.	David Watfon	14 May 1757	Colonel 23 Jan. 56
	James Biamham	do.	
	William Gieen	4 Jan. 1758	
	Mathew Dixon	do.	
	William Evies	do.	Major 7 Jan. 56
	George Moirifon	do	
	John Archer	do.	
	George Wefton	do.	
	Haity Gordon	do.	
Engineer extraordinary as Captain Lieutenant.	John Brewfe	4 Jan. 1758	
	Hugh Delbeig	do.	
	John Bugh	do.	
	William Bontein	do.	
	Richard Dawfon	do.	
	Richaid Dudgeon	do.	
	C Hubert Heniot	do.	Captain 8 Nov. 56
	Thomas Walker	do.	
	Adam Williamfon	do.	
Sub-Engineer as Lieutenant.	Thomas Sowers	4 Jan. 1758	
	Thomas Wilkinfon	do.	9 Oct. 1757
	John Williams	do.	1 Mar. 1756
	George Garth	do.	
	John Phipps	do.	
	William Spry	do.	
Practitioner Engineer as Enfign.			7 Sept. 1757
	William Dundas	14 May 1757	Lieut. 25 Aug. 56
	Rob. George Bruce	do.	eut 14 May 57
	Auguftus Deirford	do.	eut. 4 Jan. 56
	David Dundas	do.	ut. 3 Jn 56
	Thomas Baffet	do.	Lieut 14 Feb. 56
	William Roy	do.	eut. 4 Jan. 56
	Charles Tarrant	do.	eut. 5 Sept. 56
	John Chriftian Efer	do.	Lieut. 6 Dec. 57
	Richard Muller	8 Feb. 1758	
	Theophilus Lefanue	do.	
	Archibald Campbell	do.	
	Robert Morfe	do.	24 Sept. 1757
	Patrick Rofs	19 May	8 Jan. 1757
	John Montiefor	do.	Lieut. 4 July 55

Rank in the

Four Companies at NEW YORK.

Rank	Name.	Company.	Army
Captain — —	William Ogilvie	16 Apr 1757	
Lieutenant —	Lewis Pavey	31 Aug. 1747	
	Alex Colhoun	25 May 1755	
	John Rowan	20 Nov. 1757	
Captain — —	Charles Cruikshanks	17 Apr 1757	
Lieutenant —	John Mills	25 Feb. 1758-9	
	William Goden	25 Nov 1756	
	John Mackane	18 Apr 1757	
Captain — —	Peter Wraxell	7 Jan. 1755	
Lieutenant —	Walter Butler	25 June 1725	
	Archibald Caslave	Dec 17 6	
	Henry Farrent	2 M . 1758	
Captain — —	Horatio Gates	13 Sept 1754	
Lieutenant —	William Spence	16 Aug 1750	
	Arch. Mont. Brown	22 Aug. 1755	
	Richard Miller	17 Dec 1751	
Chaplain — —	James Orem	25 June 1737	
Surgeon — —	Richard Shuckburgh	do.	
	Alexander Colhoun	do	
Adjutant — —	Arch. Mont. Brown	15 Jan. 1756	

Agent, Mr Calcraft

Three Companies at SOUTH CAROLINA.

Captain — —	Thomas Goldsmith	5 May 1756	
Lieutenant —	Robert Howarth	26 Mar 1744	
	Walter Outerbridge	26 Sept. 1754	
Ensign — —	Lachlan Muntosh	25 Dec. 1750	
Captain — —	Raymond Dearcié	31 Jan 1741-2	
Lieutenant —	William Shadfole	26 Sept 1754	
	Lachlan Shaw	25 Nov. 1754	
Ensign — —	John Bogges	5 May 1755	
Captain — —	Paul Demeré	26 June 1754	
Lieutenant —	John Grey	13 Sept. 1756	
	Charles Taylor	5 Nov 1756	
Ensign — —	Richard Coytmore	20 Sept. 1754	
Surgeon — —	George Milligen	22 Jan. 1755	

Agent, Mr. Calcraft

One Company in the BAHAMA ISLANDS.

Captain — —	John Tinker	4 Apr. 1744	
Lieutenant —	John Coohin	22 Jan. 1754	
	William Massey	24 July 1754	
	Thomas McManus	20 June 1758	
Chaplain — —	Thomas Coren	21 1 . 1756	
Surgeon — —	Robert Stewart	5 May 1758	

Agent, Mr. Baker, King's-Square-Court, Soho

One Company at BERMUDAS

Captain — —	William Popple	17 Nov. 1744	
Lieutenant —	Simon Parker	26 Sept 1754	
Ensign — —	Robert Clarke	13 Nov 1755	

Agent, Mr. Mathias, Scotland-Yard.

130 COMPANIES of MARINES.

	Rank in the	
	Marines.	Army

COLONELS.

	Marines	Army
James Paterson	19 Dec. 1755	
Theodore Dury	6 Apr. 1 50	

LIEUT COLONELS

Richard Bradvihe	19 Dec. 1755	
James Burleigh	22 Apr. 1758	

MAJORS.

Hector Boisrond	9 Dec. 1755	
John Mackenzie	10 do	
John Purcell Kempe	11 do	
Samuel Boucher	20 do.	
Edward Ryenut	10 June 1756	
John Tufton Mason	20 Feb. 1758	

CAPTAINS.

		Marines	Army
2	Gabriel Sediere	5 Feb. 1755	24 Mar 1740-1
4	Charles Repington	7 do.	22 Apr. 1741
10	Thomas Dawes	13 do.	14 May 1744
12	Thomas Sheldon	15 do.	27 Sept 1745
19	John Campbell	22 do.	17 May 1748
20	Claudius Hamilton	23 do.	
21	John Bell	24 do.	
24	Thomas Wightwick	27 do.	
29	Samuel Prosser	4 Mu.	
31	Alexander Irons	6 do.	
34	Richard Brough	9 do.	
35	Henry Smith	10 do.	
42	John Johnston	11 do.	
37	Christopher Gauntlett	13 do	
38	Arthur Tooker Collins	14 do	
39	Walter Caruthers	15 do	
40	John Vere	16 do	
44	Richard Hawkins	19 do	
47	Robert Burdett	22 do	
48	John Yeo	23 do	
46	Walter Johnstone	31 May	2 Jan. 1749-50
17	Alexander Ogilvie	17 July	
51	George Thomas	25 Nov	9 June 1740
54	Hon James Forbes	25 do.	24 Aug. 1745
55	Daniel Campbell	26 do.	
56	Dudley Crofts	27 do	
13	James Tichborne	28 do.	
57	George Langley	29 do.	
59	Alexander Cathcart	2 Dec	
5	William Billing	do.	
60	Francis Hay	3 do	
42	Thomas Marriott	do.	43 Joseph

CAPTAINS.

43	Joseph Austin	3 Dec 1755	26	Griffith Williams	19 Aug 1756
53	Donald McDonald	6 do.	83	William Wetherston	15 Feb. 57
61	John Sutter	7 do.	108	David Hepburn	19 do.
62	Edward Howarth	8 do.	130	Thomas Piele	20 do.
63	Robert Douglas	9 do.	107	Robert Douglas	21 do.
64	James Murray	10 do.	23	Thomas Backhouse	22 do.
65	Thomas Buckston	11 do.	103	Saxton Convers	23 do.
67	John Brown	13 do.	6	William Fulton	24 do.
68	Colin Campbell	14 do.	100	John Flood	25 do.
1	Archibald Campbell	15 do.	101	Stephen Newnson	26 do.
69	Robert Bird	15 do.	105	Erskine M'Ferzie	27 do.
3	George Ord	15 do.	106	Charles Templeman	28 do.
70	Samuel Culbeck	15 do.	110	Robert Morris	1 Mar.
71	John Martin	17 do.	15	John Nugent	2 do.
72	Lancelot Willan	18 do.	113	John Mackey	3 do.
74	George Biggs	20 do.	119	Francis Napier	5 do.
75	Jacob Lonsdale	21 do.	118	Robert Cotton	6 do.
76	Edward Kyffin	22 do.	117	Hon. Francis Leslie	7 do.
77	Richard Dennison	23 do.	120	John Hughes	9 do.
73	John Barnwell Waller	25 do.	125	Horatio Gary	10 do.
36	Charles Bay...	5 June 1756	123	Robert Barker	11 do.
45	James Wilder	5 do.	121	William North	13 do.
41	George Cockburne	do.	124	William Lloyd	13 do.
89	William Davidson	6 do.	128	Richard Weston	15 do.
16	John Pitcairn	8 do.	111	Robert Rooke	17 do.
81	† John Goodenough	16 do.	127	John Graham	18 do.
82	Gardner Bulstrode	17 do.	115	Richard Gardner	20 do.
33	William Bolton	do.	109	Hon. J. Maitland	22 do.
84	James Short	19 do.	114	Alexander Trotter	23 do.
85	John Pozer	21 do.	129	Edward M'Poore	24 do.
85	William Douglas	22 do.	112	William Verner	25 do.
89	Dennis Bond	23 do.	99	Benjamin Leaper	10 June
92	Thomas Troy	24 do.	66	Joshua Stone	4 Sept.
83	William Thompson	25 do.	126	Harrie Innes	5 do.
91	John Elliot	26 do.	116	Hon. Hugh Sempill	16 Nov.
94	Ralph Teesdale	28 do.	7	Stawell Chudleigh	15 Apr. 58
95	Robert Shirley	29 do.	22	Turbil Wainwright	16 do.
90	Daniel Campbell	30 do.	8	Robert Walsh	17 do.
97	William Lutman	1 July	78	John Chalmers	18 do.
96	Thomas Wight	2 do.	58	Lawrence Mercer	19 do.
98	Thomas Stamper	3 do.	104	Charles Hughes	20 do.
18	Edward Farmer	6 do.	93	Thomas Davis	21 do.
27	George Manley	19 do.	11	William Souter	22 do.
50	Styles Ravenscroft	21 do.			
30	Sir William Wescombe	22 do.			
25	Henry Gore	22 do.			
49	John Tupper	16 Aug.			
72	John Blinkhorne	17 do.			
32	Charles Fletcher	18 do.			

† } Rank in the Army { 25 Oct. 1744
† } { 17 Feb. 1745-6
‡ } { 17 Jan. 1746-7

T 2   FIRST

Marines.

FIRST LIEUTENANTS.

26	Geo. Dannet	1 Mar. 1755	13	John Bowater	21 July 56
29	George Galton	4 do.	9	Roger Richardson	22 do.
34	James Jenkins	9 do.	17	Thomas Avarne	23 do.
54	Richard Mompesson	2 Dec.	48	James Kirk	18 Aug.
59	William Sadler	7 do.	55	Thomas P. Peel	19 do.
66	Peter Livingston	14 do.	41	Hugh Frazer	20 do.
65	Thornhill Heathcote	15 do.	73	John Bree	21 do.
68	William Nethersole	17 do	75	John Caton	22 do.
71	Mark Shaftoe	20 do	14	John Smith	10 Sept.
73	John Barber	22 do.	85	William Grosvenor	28 Oct.
77	Joseph Galton	26 do.	8	John Purves	17 Feb. 1757
79	Thadday le Charter	28 do.	37	John Riddsale	18 do
82	George Stuckey	29 do.	25	John Knox	19 do.
10	James Walsh	do	40	Alexander Ross	20 do.
15	John Shuter	30 do	4	Roger Stevenson	21 do.
45	Thomas Grant	7 June 1756	111	Henry Walter	22 do.
30	Maurice Wemys	8 do.	28	Robert Cahan	23 do.
20	George Wade	9 do.	96	William Vario	24 do.
50	Charles Champion	10 do.	101	Thomas Timms	25 do.
83	John Hayes	10 do	103	Samuel Mitchell	26 do.
58	Thomas Astbury	11 do.	104	Christopher Middleton	27 do.
86	John M'Fie	do.	105	Miles Sandys	28 do.
89	Charles Mackay	13 do.	110	Joseph Bushell	1 Mar.
92	Joseph Smith	14 do	114	Thomas Allen	2 do.
84	William Rotheram	16 do.	109	Dudley Loftus	3 do.
88	Thomas Groves	17 do.	113	William Douglas	4 do.
91	William Douglas	18 do	117	Reginald Graham	5 do.
93	Arthur Bridge	20 do.	81	William Burgh	6 do.
100	William Lewis	22 do.	120	Samuel Davis	7 do.
97	Mordecai Abbot	23 do	112	Edward O Neale	8 do.
90	George Innes	24 do.	118	William Sabine	do.
98	Lele Brown	26 do.	51	Christopher Zobell	9 do.
99	Robert Kennedy	27 do	116	Olive Kelly	do.
42	Andrew Elliot	29 do.	115	John Burt	10 do.
44	Charles Frazer	30 do.	122	Richard Brady	do.
46	John Campbell	1 July	119	Arthur Good	11 do.
1	Archibald Campbell	2 do.	53	William Burgess	12 do.
49	Alexander Campbell	3 do.	56	Robert Myston	do.
24	Henry Fletcher	5 do	69	Towry Phillips	13 do.
38	William Forde	6 do.	57	James Cassidy	do.
39	William Johnston	7 do	6	George Bader	14 do.
18	George Preston	8 do.	124	James Mowbray	14 do.
19	George Logan	9 do.	102	William Robertson	15 do.
21	William Harding	10 do.	123	Samuel Hadley	15 do.
22	Robert Rochead	11 do.	108	John M'Leod	16 do.
77	William Forster	12 do	52	Thomas Crawford	16 do.
11	John Barclay	12 do	2	James Brown	17 do.
31	John Mackay	13 do.	94	William Lock	17 do.
32	Duncan Munro	14 do.	76	George Elliott	18 do.
35	John Graham	15 do	7	Benjamin Adair	18 do.
36	Coin Graham	16 do.	130	William Caunter	19 do.
12	Walter Steuart	17 do.			126 Thomas

* Rank in the Army, 11 Sept. 1745.

FIRST LIEUTENANTS.

126	Thomas Hamilton	19 Mai 1757	64	Barnabas Banks	10 June 1757
67	T Thorpe Fowke	20 do.	62	William Bowler	4 Oct.
106	Ben Jenkinson	do.	65	John Chambers	5 do.
125	Samuel Kemp	21 do.	9	Thomas Wells	6 do.
43	Thomas Bell	21 do	82	David Watfon	14 Apr 1758
128	William Cawthorne	22 do.	60	Patrick Hamilton	15 do.
74	Thomas Felster	22 do.	47	John M Intyre	16 do.
107	Charles Chandlis	23 do.	61	William Nefbit	17 do.
52	John Cairns	24 do.	63	Jonathan Dales	18 do.
127	John Brown	do.	70	James Fowler	19 do
21	Harvey Fleming	25 do.	72	Robert Emott	20 do.
123	Richard Devins	21 Apr.	5	John Burgh	21 do.
87	John Rowell	9 June	16	William Bowers	22 do.

SECOND LIEUTENANTS.

11	Edward Horney	14 Feb. 1755	64	Nathan James	1 Jan. 1756
31	James Gardiner	12 Nov	78	Peter Great	do.
43	John Monro	17 do.	79	Alexander Small	2 do.
3	Thomas Kirvey	27 do.	80	William Harman	3 do.
8	Jeremiah Broomer	22 do.	27	Stephen Davis	4 do.
71	William Sharp	25 do.	4	Thomas Biggs	6 do.
73	James Cleland	27 do.	5	William Downes	7 do
76	John Bofwell	30 do.	6	William Cooper	8 do.
77	David Wilkie	1 Dec.	18	Charles Tucker	27 May
78	John Fownes	2 do.	32	James Cuming	28 do.
79	Francis Lindfey	3 do.	76	Peter Penfold	30 do.
80	Charles Sheare	4 do.	63	Thomas Birnall	31 do.
51	Thomas Wood	5 do	1	Samuel Stratham	1 June
52	Archibald Douglas	6 do	25	John Dalton	3 do.
54	John Duffe	8 do.	23	Thomas Nightingale	7 do.
56	Colin Campbell	10 do.	22	Richard Libberd	9 do.
57	Robert Hope	11 do	17	Samuel Casket	10 do.
59	Onefipherus Swan	13 do.	15	Robert Scott	11 do.
60	Thomas Arnott	15 do.	63	John Hardy	12 do.
62	Hector M‘Neale	16 do.	82	Hon James Rollo	14 do.
63	Robert Mollicon	17 do.	100	Chriftopher Allot	15 do.
64	——— Sinclair	18 do.	86	Robert Rois	17 do.
65	William Maxwell	19 do	18	William Patterfon	19 do.
66	Arthur Walker	20 do	89	John Hadden	20 do.
67	Duncan Campbell	21 do.	92	Jofeph Lingford	21 do.
70	Patrick Barclay	24 do	64	Thomas Mint	22 do.
71	William Jackfon	25 do	65	William Baldwin	20 do.
72	William Horfbergh	26 do.	96	Richard Bers	27 do.
73	John Raymond	27 do	98	John Mercer	29 do.
74	William Firnie	28 do.	99	James Dawes	30 do.
75	James Larnet	29 do	82	Robert Coddington	3 July
77	John Sinclair	31 do.	86	Thomas Price	do.
					St David

6 ⎫
7 ⎬ Rank in the Army ⎰ 1st 4 July 1742
4 ⎭ ⎱ 26 Feb 1755-6

SECOND LIEUTENANTS.

No.	Name	Date	No.	Name	Date
85	Edward Herbert	6 July 1756	35	Theoph. Boisfrond	26 Oct 1756
87	Laurence O'Farrell	8 do.	47	John Chriftian	27 do.
88	John Woodruff	9 do.	22	John Jeffeys	28 do.
91	John Lloyd	11 do.	85	Francis Stuart	17 Feb 57
92	William Elliot	12 do.	81	David Cuming	17 do.
94	Ja. Berckenhout	13 do.	89	Alpine Grant	17 do.
41	Jeffe Adair	do.	38	Stuart Robinson	18 do.
96	Walfingh. Dowdefwell	14 do	69	George Forbes	do.
42	William Span	do.	28	Alexander Byre	do.
99	Colin Campbell	15 do.	45	Robert Lloyd	do.
93	Francis Burk	16 do.	37	James Anderfon.	do
46	William Nicholls	do.	3	David Johnston	do.
97	John Fitzfimons	17 do.	93	Robert Burton	20 do
100	John Gray	18 do.	39	Harry Gordon	21 do.
47	Donald M'Donald	19 do.	9	J Huntf Branson	do.
90	Charles Chalmers	20 do.	112	Lancelot Rutter	22 do.
95	Richard Timpson	21 do.	26	James Coil	do.
34	John Thomfon	do	4	Robert M'Leod	do.
22	Alexander Lyon	22 do.	6	Leefon Paterfon	23 do.
5	James Gray	do	7	William Pritchard	do.
18	John Roberts	23 do.	14	Alexander Hume	do
20	Richard Bifhop	24 do.	102	Bartholomew Chaundy	24 do.
21	Boteler Harris	25 do	102	Richard Lloyd	do.
24	Thomas Campbell	26 do.	103	Thomas Hodgfon	25 do.
38	Thomas Hardyman	29 do.	101	Andrew Nicholfon	26 do.
34	Edward Owen	30 do	105	Archibald Forreft	do.
46	Manners Lifle	1 Aug.	104	William Huckell	26 do.
2	Francis Hill	2 do	101	John Ogilvy	27 do.
6	John Sylvefter	3 do.	106	Andrew Erfkine	do.
9	James Urquhart	4 do.	107	Arthur Buttle	do.
16	Ebenezer Kirkpatrick	5 do.	108	Richard Steele	28 do.
17	Charles Bell	6 do.	109	Jofhua Howell	do.
18	James Campbell	7 do.	110	James Mafon	do.
49	Thomas Morgan	9 do,	111	Alexander Stuart	1 Mar.
24	John Trail	11 do	112	John Fieldhoufe	do.
37	James Johnfton	14 do.	106	Jofeph Baines	do.
28	John Green	15 do.	107	Hugh Higgins	2 do.
29	Alexander M'Leod	16 do.	109	Jofhua Thornton	2 do.
69	Thomas Negus	do	110	William Conyers	3 do.
67	John Peck	17 do	111	William Hayes	do
30	William Price	do.	26	Bartholomew Williams	4 do.
58	Daniel Belt	18 do.	23	Thomas Holland	do.
33	Arch. Simpfon	19 do.	10	Thomas Loake	do.
63	Stephen Nevinfon	do.	11	Walter Paterfon	do
35	John Wilkinfon	21 do.	12	Alexander M'Donald	5 do.
36	John Macartney	22 do	61	William Anderfon	do
27	James M'Donald	23 do	13	James Green	do.
12	Alex Livingfton	19 Oct.	17	David Coutes	6 do.
53	R. Coffen Blankley	20 do.	51	Nathaniel English	do.
14	Stephen Ellis	21 do.	53	John Mihil	7 do
40	Thomas Gozna	22 do	54	Grant Home	do.
50	William Cox	24 do.	55	John France	do.

59 Robert

SECOND LIEUTENANTS

No.	Name	Date	No.	Name	Date
59	Robert Wilkers	8 Mar. 1757	43	George Clerk	30 Mar. 1757
65	Daniel McLeod	do	1	Thomas Grifith	1 Apr.
39	Francis Waldton	9 do	44	Stephen Page	2 do.
29	John Halsted	do	72	Brent Moore	21 do.
20	Thomas Sterling	do	55	Vincent Down	9 June
130	Charles Jackman	10 do	15	Enye Allen Wood	10 do.
126	Bryan Gray	do	44	Thomas Capps	11 do.
128	Archbald ...	11 do	65	John Allen	12 do.
113	Thomas Evcott	do	31	William Fyfield	14 do.
114	John McMillan	do	117	John Hunt	25 do.
116	John Maffle	12 do	105	Edward Gregg	3 Oct.
116	Peter Bachan	do	22	Thomas Sneyd	5 do.
117	Wm B Biggs	do	21	Ralph Barker	6 do.
118	Robert Man	13 do	63	Henry Wren	7 do
119	Samuel Anderson	do	70	David Ogilvie	8 do.
118	John Walker	14 do	81	James Hay	9 do.
119	William Mitchill	do	74	Abraham Wotton	10 do.
124	Colin Campbell	do	91	Isaac Bche ...	26 Mar. 1758
124	John Campbell	15 do	127	William Walker	27 do.
92	James Campbell	do	19	Gordon	28 do.
34	Alexander Campbell	do	31	Aaron Darby	29 do.
120	John Bell	16 do	43	Joseph Conway	30 do.
120	Robert Allen	do	57	Henry Head	31 do.
121	John Savage	do	104	Alexander Brown	1 Apr.
128	John Fletcher	17 do	8	P M.	2 do.
7	Thomas Green	do	52	Thomas Hayward	3 do.
62	James Cathcart	do	19	Joseph Adams	4 do.
129	Thomas Gregg	18 do	157	George Willoughby	5 do.
50	George Henry Kyffin	19 do	130	Singleton Rochfort	6 do.
121	John Paul	19 do	113	Joseph Hazlewood	7 do
122	James Knox	20 do	125	William Cooper	8 do.
123	Charles Von Rull	21 do	122	Thomas Barclay	9 do.
124	Thomas McBrair	do	25	William Dancer	10 do.
125	Evan Cameron	do	103	John Willis	11 do.
60	Mat Pop Manby	22 do	15	Thomas Spooner	12 do.
120	John Redsy	do	91	George Phelps	13 do.
49	William Graham	23 do	15	Francis Ward	14 do.
114	Francis Moore	24 do	53	Charles Coalthest	15 do.
115	John Churchward	do	61	Robert Gardiner	16 do.
114	William Atkinson	25 do	15	James Stuart	17 do.
2	Richard Pulford	do	84	John Baggs	18 do.
36	Archibald Douglas	26 do	93	John Stretch	19 do.
30	Edward Thompson	27 do	103	John Kent	20 do.
40	Edward Wall	28 do	129	George Martin	21 do.
41	George Nairn	29 do	87	John Beady	22 do.

ADJUTANTS

Ch John Hardy 1 Aug 1756 — P Samuel Mitchell 2 Apr. 1758
Po Thomas Grant 24 Aug. 1756 — P Charles Darby do.
Ply John Chicken 10 June 1757 — Po Colin Campbell do.
Ch John Hadden 2 Apr. 1758

QUARTER MASTERS.

Po Peter Livingston 1 ... 1750 — C William Walker 1 Aug 1756

		Rank in the	
Six Companies at Plymouth			
Park.	*Name.*	*Corps.*	*Army.*
Captain - -	John ... Gapin	16 Dec. 17..	
Lieutenant	J.	26 J.... ...	
Ensign - -	S...d ...	2. ... 1 .7	
Captain - -	P...ro, ...	... 1.5..	
Lieutenant -	Jo.. W.......	2. ...	Capt. 13 Mar. 1742
Ensign - -	... Good	2 Fr.. .. o .5	
Captain - -	Henry Keen	5 July 1755	2. July 1755
Lieutenant -	W.. ... Loyd	12 Nov. 1757	1. Mar. 17.7
Ensign - -	William O... ..	.. July 1751	
Captain - -	William Catherwood	16 Jan. 1752	17 Feb. 1746
Lieutenant -	Benjamin Sladden	21 Jan. 1737-8	
Ensign - -	Roger Dalling	22 Mar. 1757	
Captain - -	Richard Corbett	10 Feb. 1753	23 July 1743
Lieutenant -	Boyle Burton	22 Mar. 1757	
Ensign - -	Ray	7 Apr. 1758	
Captain - -	William Williams	22 Jan. 1754	23 Jan. 1741
Lieutenant -	Enos Dexter	12 Feb. 1750-1	26 Apr. 1741
Ensign - -	Adam Gordon	1 Dec. 1757	
Surgeon -	William Lake	13 Nov. 1756	
Five Companies at GUERNSEY.			
Captain - -	James Johnstone	11 Jan. 1758	1. Nov. 1746
Lieutenant -	James Maxwell	17 Apr. 1755	
Ensign - -	John Higgers	18 June 1757	
Captain - -	John Windus	. Aug. 1749	10 May 1740
Lieutenant -	George Ballard	29 July 1757	
Ensign - -	George Hawley	8 July 1757	
Captain - -	William Blackett	1 Mar. 1758	Major 22 Nov. 56
Lieutenant -	Lewis Oury	8 Oct. 172.	
Ensign - -	HopeLong Tidcomb	23 July 17.8	
Captain -	Lucy Wesson	21 Jan. 17.8	13 Feb. 1748
Lieutenant -	Benedict Blogden	2 Nov. 1733	
Ensign - -	John Mar... d	28 June 1751	
Captain - -	Lt. John Mylne Et.	10 May 17..	29 Nov. 1745
Lieutenant -	Gallian Maclean	8 July 1757	
Ensign - - -	John Jenkinson	8 July 1757	
Four Companies at HULL.			
Captain - -	Thomas Shadwell	4 Sept. 1745	7 May 1711
Lieutenant -	Henry Watkins	13 Jan. 1753	13 Jan. 1753
Ensign - -	Joseph Beach	5 Jan. 1747-8	
Captain - -	John Lind	12 Nov. 1757	Major 28 Nov. 1757
Lieutenant -	Charles Parkinson	1 Nov. 1739	
Ensign - - - -	Richard Hargrave	22 Mar. 1757	
Captain - -	James Edmonds	27 Jan. 1753	3 Jan. 1750
Lieutenant -	John Snell	16 Jan. 1754	. May 1754
Ensign - -	Thomas Walker	2 Feb. 1754	
Captain - -	Charles Draper	5 Jan. 1754	
Lieutenant -	Charles Healey	8 Feb. 1737-8	
Ensign - -	Anthony Renwick	12 Feb. 1741-3	

			Rank in the
			Army.
Rank.	Name.	Company.	

Two Companies at CHESTER.

Captain - -	William Taylor	22 Aug. 1744	12 Jan. 1740
Lieutenant -	Joseph Winder	5 Apr. 1757	13 Sept. 1754
Ensign - -	Robert Pullen	11 Oct. 1748	
Captain - -	James Draper	13 Mar. 49-50	19 June 1734
Lieutenant -	Hugh Lloyd	24 July 1756	13 Nov. 1755
Ensign - -	Charles Turner	5 Aug. 1731	

Two Companies at TILBURY FORT.

Captain - -	Francis Cylian	25 Mar. 1744	5 July 1755
Lieutenant -	James Parker	9 Aug. 1756	22 Apr. 1755
Ensign - - -	Walter Ogilvie	5 June 1758	
Captain - -	John Lovell	24 Nov. 1748	28 Aug. 1737
Lieutenant - -	Richard Hicks	17 Nov. 1746	
Ensign - - -	Philip Foley	13 Oct. 1755	

One Company at TINMOUTH.

Captain - -	Thomas Middleton	19 Apr. 1742	
Lieutenant -	Ralph Smith	17 Mar. 49-50	
Ensign - -	Charles Nethercott	10 Nov. 1749	7 Aug. 1746

One Company at LANDGUARD-FORT.

Captain - -	George Coote	8 Nov. 1756	20 Oct. 1746
Lieutenant -	George Hammond	12 Feb. 1755	
Ensign - -	Robert Bruce	20 Nov. 1750	17 Feb. 1746

One Company at PENDENNIS.

Captain - -	Mathew Sewell	24 July 1754	Lieut. Col. 4 Oct. 45
Lieutenant -	Geo Lew: Hamilton	10 Mar. 1753	
Ensign - -	John Scotton	9 Aug. 1757	

One Company at SCILLY.

Captain - -	Charles Jefferyson	21 Jan. 1737-8	23 Aug. 1711
Lieutenant -	John Sherwin	8 July 1757	
Ensign - -	Abraham Mills	do.	

Agent. Mr. Fauve, Pultney-Street.

Four Companies in IRELAND.

Captain - -	William Cosby	22 Nov. 1756
1st Lieutenant	John Plukenett	3 Nov. 1757
2d Lieutenant	James Whittle	22 Nov. 1756
Ensign - -	Morrison	do.
Captain - -	Robert Barton	4 Jan. 1757
1st Lieutenant	Hugh Massey	22 Nov. 1756
2d Lieutenant	Henry Ross Gaven	do.
Ensign - -	John Higgins	do.
Captain - -	Stewart	22 Nov. 1756
1st Lieutenant	John Warren	do.
2d Lieutenant	Finney	do.
Ensign - -	Henry Snow	27 Aug. 1757
Captain - -	Robert Jephson	22 Nov. 1756
1st Lieutenant	Arthur Blennerhassett	do.
2d Lieutenant	Edward Bignel	
Ensign - -	John Campbell	

Garrifon.	Rank.	Officers Names.	Per Annum.
Berwick - -	Governor	Lt. Gen John Guife	600 0 0
	Lieutenant Governor	Hon Col J. Barrington	182 10 0
	Town Major	Enfign Samuel Rogers	73 0 0
	Town Adjutant	George Douglas	73 0 0
	Chaplain	William Siffon	121 13 4
	Surgeon	James Wood	45 12 6
Blacknefs-Caftle	Governor	Hon. Charles Hope Weir	300 0 0
	Lieutenant	John Stuart	73 0 0
Calfhot - -	Governor	William Knapton	45 12 6
Carlifle - -	Governor	Colonel John Stanwix	182 10 0
	Lieutenant Governor	Captain C. Defcloyfeaux	182 10 0
	Town Major	Lieutenant John Cliffe	73 0 0
Chefter - -	Governor	M Gl. G. Earl Cholmondeley	182 10 0
	Lieut. Governor	Hon. L. Gl. Ja. Cholmondeley	182 10 0
Cinque Ports -	Lord Warden	Lionel *Duke of* Dorfet	500 0 0
	Lieut. Dover Caftle	Sir Thomas Hales	182 10 0
	Deputy Lieutenant {	Thomas Broadley Richard Roufe }	109 10 0
	Chaplain	John Minet	36 10 0
Dunbarton Caftle	Governor	*Earl of* Caffilles	300 0 0
	Lieutenant Governor	John Leman }	182 10 0
	Lieutenant	John Leman }	
	Enfign	Archibald M'Corkell	54 15 0
Dartmouth --	Governor	Arthur Holdfworth	182 10 0
	Fort Major	Thomas Palmer	73 0 0
Edinburgh --	Governor	Lt. Gl. Humphry Bland	300 0 0
	Lieutenant Governor	Richard Coren	182 10 0
	Fort Major	George Whitemore	91 5 0
	Lieutenant {	George Whitemore	73 0 0
		David Kinloch	73 0 0
	Enfign	Jofeph Roberton	54 15 0
	Chaplain	William Haig	45 12 6
	Surgeon	John Gardner	45 12 6
Gravefend and Tilbury	Governor	Lt. Gl C Ld. Cadogan	300 0 0
	Lieutenant Governor	Charles Whitworth	182 10 0
	Fort Major	Captain John Lovell	73 0 0
	Chaplain	James How	36 10 0
	Surgeon	John How	45 12 6
Guernfey - --	Governor	Lt. Gen. Lord De Lawarr	0 0 0
	Lieutenant Governor	Capt. Sir John Mylne Bt.	182 10 0
	Chaplain	John Le Mefurier	121 13 4

Garrifons.

Garrison.	Rank.	Officers Names.	Per Annum.		
Hull	Governor	L. Gen. Harry Pu_ney	600	0	0
	Lieutenant Governor	M. G. Ld Rob. Manners	182	10	0
	Town Major	Ensign Richard Hargrave	7_	0	0
	Chaplain	John Clark	121	13	4
	Surgeon	——— Melling	4_	12	6
Hurst-Castle	Governor	Sir Henry Bellenden	182	10	0
Fort George near Inverness	Governor	L. G. Sir Charles Howard	500	0	0
	Deputy Governor	Major William Caulfield	300	0	0
	Fort Adjutant	Humphry Colquhoun	73	0	0
	Surgeon	Alexander Monro	109	10	0
Jersey	Governor	L. General John Huske	0	0	0
	Lieutenant Governor	Capt. Geo Collingwood	182	10	0
	Fort Major and Adj.	Alexander Hogge	85	3	4
	Chaplain	Francis Payne	36	10	0
Landguard Fort	Governor	M G Ld Geo Beauclerck	365	0	0
	Lieutenant Governor	Philip Thi_nette	182	10	0
	Chaplain	John Loyde	36	10	0
St. Maws	Captain or Keeper	M Gen Alex Duroure	109	10	0
	Deputy Governor	Arthur Kemp	45	12	6
Pendennis-Castle	Governor	Lt. Colonel Arthur Owen	300	0	0
	Lieutenant Governor	Major Richard Bowles	91	5	0
Plymouth	Governor	John Vi_ Ligonier F. M.	1289	2	6
	Lieutenant Governor	Lieutenant John Williams	182	10	0
	Fort Major	Lieutenant William Joyce	73	0	0
	Chaplain	John Corham Hoxham	121	13	4
Portland Castle	Governor	Thomas Gollop	91	5	0
Portsmouth	Governor	L. General Henry Hawley	700	0	0
	Lieutenant Governor	Capt John Ma_ras	182	10	0
	Town Major	Ensign Patrick Douglas	73	0	0
	Town Adjutant	Capt Charles D_averant	91	5	0
	Chaplain	Henry Robinson	121	13	_
	Physician	George Cuthbert	182	10	0
	Surgeon	Edward Lindzee	45	12	6
South Sea Castle	Deputy Governor	Nathaniel Smith	91	5	0
Sheerness	Governor	L. G. S. John Mordaunt	500	0	0
	Lieutenant Governor	Major Henry Hut_	182	10	0
	Fort Major	John Young	73	0	0
	Chaplain	Theodore de la F_	36	10	0
	Surgeon	William Hicks	45	12	0
Scilly-Island	Governor	Francis Ea_l Godol_in	0	0	0
	Lieutenant Governor	Hon. M. G. Geo Bo_awen	1_2	10	0
	Surgeon	James _io_	45	12	0
Scarb. Castle	Governor	_o_n_	16	0	0
Stirling Castle	Governor	L. C. J. _arl of Loudoun	300	0	0
	Deputy Governor	M G James Abercromby	182	10	0
	Major	David Cun_ _on	91	5	0
	Lieutenant	{ David Cunningham	_3	0	0
		{ Charles F'p__on	_3	0	0
	Ensign	John Napie_	54	15	0
	Chaplain	William Campbell	_	12	6

U 2   Ca___

Garrison.	Rank.	Officers Names	Per Annum.
Clif Fort near	Governor —	M G. S. And Agnew Bt.	300 0 0
Tinmouth	Lieut. Governor	Thomas Lacey —	182 10 0
Upnor —	Governor —	L Col. William Deane	182 10 0
Tower of London {	Constable —	Cha Ea. Cornwallis	1000 0 0
	Lieutenant —	L C. I C M. of Winchester	700 0 0
	Dep Lieutenant	Charles Rainsford	365 0 0
	Tower Major —	Ma o Ch Hen Colins —	182 10 0
	Chaplain —	Edward Horby - —	121 13 4
	Gentleman Porter	Sir Thomas J'Anson —	84 6 8
	Gentleman Gealer	Thomas Scott - —	70 0 0
	Physician —	Caleb Hardinge - —	182 10 0
	Surgeon —	Lewis Davis — —	45 12 6
	Apothecary —	Richard Jaques —	10 0 0
Fort William {	Governor —	Hon L Gen. Rich Onslow	300 0 0
	Dep Governor	L Col John Leighton —	182 10 0
Fort Augustus {	Governor —	Hon Lt G. Sr Ch Howard	0 0 0
	Dep Governor —	Alexander Trapaud —	300 0 0
	Fort Adjutant	Richard Trought —	73 0 0
Windsor {	Governor —	Geo E of Cardigan	1182 10 0
	Lieut Governor	Hon Col T Brudenell —	182 10 0
No. Yarmouth	Governor —	Hon Roger Townshend	102 10 0
Isle of Wight {	Governor —	J E of Portsmouth —	500 0 0
	Lieut Governor	M G. Henry Holmes —	305 0 0
	Sandown Fort	John Leigh — —	45 12 6
	Yarmouth Castle	John Burrard — —	102 10 0
	Carisbrook Castle	Lr G. Mau Eocland —	182 10 0
	Cowes Castle —	Robert Grylls — —	182 10 0
St. James's Park	Master Gunner —	James Deal — —	36 10 0

Officers of the Garrison of *Gibraltar*.

Governor —	William Earl Home	730 0 0
Lieut. Governor -	Col T. Dunb. —	730 0 0
Com of Stores, &c. ·	Lord Erskine —	547 10 0
Chap. to the Gov.	John Chalmers —	121 13 4
Secre. to the Gov -	Richard Dacre —	182 10 0
Dep Judg. Advo.	Hew Craig —	182 10 0
Town Major - -	Maj David Chapeau	91 5 0
Town Adjutant -	John Tyrell —	54 15 0
Surgeon Major -	Arthur Baines —	182 10 0
Mates - - - {	John Stone — —	91 5 0
	William Dogvell	91 5 0
Provost Marsh. -	John Peck —	73 0 0
Gaol Man - -	Richard Dacre —	18 5 0
Porter - - -	Jeremiah Beeman	18 5 0

Officers

Officers in the Plantations on the Military Establishment.

Garrisons	Ranks.	Officers Names.	Per Annum
Province of Nova-Scotia	Governor ———	Col. C. Lawrence	1000 0 0
	Lieutenant Governor	Col. R. Monckton	0 0 0
	Secretary ——	William Sheriffe ——	182 10 0
Annapolis Royal	Lieutenant Governor	Col. R. Monckton	182 10 0
	Fort Major ———	Erasmus Phillips —	73 0 0
	Clerk of Stores and Provisions }	Erasmus Phillips —	73 0 0
	Judge Advocate, &c.	William Sheriffe —	73 0 0
	Chaplain ———	Gregory Sharpe —	121 13 4
	Surgeon ———	J. Steel	54 15 0
Canso ———	Fort Major ———		73 0 0
	Clerk of Stores, &c		73 0 0
	Judge Advocate —	Robert Porter ——	73 0 0
	Chaplain ———	Henry Yong ——	121 13 4
Placentia ———	Lieutenant Governor	Otho Hamilton	182 10 0
St. John's ——	Lieutenant Governor	L. Col. John Bradstreet	82 10 0
Newfoundland	Surgeon's Mate ——	John Mower ———	45 12 6

Reduced Officers of his Majesty's Land-Forces and Marines on Half-Pay in Great-Britain.

Sir Daniel O'Carroll's Dragoons, 1712
Lieutenant Richard Lewis
Major Richard Pearce Stapleton
Earl of Ross's Dragoons, reduced 1712
Cornet Arthur Leahin
Lt. Col. Starho..'s Dragoons reduced 1712
Quarter Master James Flinn
Surgeon Peter Genest
Colonel Gorsuch's Dragoons
Cornet Lewis Rose
Quarter Master Gideon De Janies
Captain Cash
M. G. Forlack's Regiment of Dragoons 1712
Cornet Charles Kibert
B. G. Wicker's Regiment of Dragoons 1712
Captain George Hoe
Lieutenant Joseph M'Nee
Cornet Thomas Lane
Adjutant Boyle Heweton
Captain Francis La Forgere
Lieutenant D'arcy Hartwell
Cornet Daniel Cracknell
M. G. Desbride's Regiment of Dragoons 1712
Major Charles Webb
Lieutenant Joshua
Surgeon Charles

Colonel Magny's Dragoons.
Lieutenant Colonel William Vachell
Lieutenant Matthew Derry
Cornet Robert Norton
Officer Second
Cornet W. Davies
Peter de Cuala
Lieutenant Robert Hodson
Major General Gurney's Dragoons.
Officer Second
Captain G. Peter D...
Lieutenant John W...
Cornet Peter Le Clerc
.... Dragoons.
Cornet Richard Gurney
Cornet Francis Canada
Captain Edmund Okeeden, on Second
Major D. Afra's Dragoons reduced 1712
Cornet John Wiseman
B. G. Montagu's Foot reduced 1712
Lieutenant Samuel Cherry
Lieutenant Adjutant Foot reduced 1713
.... Mordaunt
Lieutenant .... reduced 1713
.... Thomas Bate
.... Enfield

B. g.

Brig. Gen. Newton'*s Foot* reduced 1713
   Captain Claude de la Vabre
Colonel Molefworth's *Foot reduced* 1713
   Lieutenant Richard St. John
          William Holcombe
Colonel Leigh's *Foot* reduced   1713
   Enfign Henry Hele
Lieut. Gen. Evans's *Foot* reduced   1713
   Surgeon George Mercer
Major Gen. Rooke's *Foot* reduced 1712
   Captain Brudenell Rooke
   Lieutenant Warnam St. Leger
   Enfign John Brozet
   Adjutant Edward Rich
Colonel Maurice Naffau's *Foot* re. 1712
   Lieutenant Robert Langford
          Thomas Holmts
   Enfign Alexander Jordan
Brig General Kane's *Foot* reduced 1713
   Captain David De Charmes
   Lieutenant John Clerck
   Enfign John Murphey
Lt. Gen. Wynne's *Foot reduced*   1712
   Enfign Francis Cuffe
Colonel Butler's *Foot reduced*   1712
   Enfign James Cromelin
Colonel Wm. Stanhope's *Foot* r. 1712
   Captain John Edwards
   Surgeon William Scott
Sir Robert Rich's *Foot*
   Lieutenant George Biffe
Sir Charles Hotham's *Foot.*
   Captain Josiah Laborde
   Captain Lieut. John Soubin
Brigadier General Stanwix's *Foot*
   Lieutenant Joseph Lawrence
          Thomas Parkinfon
          Archibald Enos
Lord Mark Kerr's *Foot*
   Lieutenant John Maitland
          James Dunlop
   Captain G. Goodwin, *en Secord*
Brig. General Munden's *Foot*
   Lieutenant Richard Hoblyn
Lieutenant General Gore's *Foot*
   Captain Robert Eeles.
Lieutenant General Tyrrell's *Foot*
   Lieutenant William Minors
          Peter Ducla
Brig. General Dubourgay's *Foot*
   Lieutenant David Guilhien

Lord Slane's *Foot*
   Lieutenant Henry Brightman
          Lancelot Dawes
   Enfign John Fountaine
Lieutenant General Fielding's *Foot*
   Lieutenant Henry Gayer
   Enfign Roger Griffith
Brigadier General Jones's *Foot*
   Enfign Thomas De Renzy
Lieutenant General Dalzell's *Foot*
   Lt. Colonel Daniel Heiing *as Captain*
Major-General Vezey's *Foot*
   Captain Peter Scale
   Lieutenant Lewis Delaftang
          Daniel Canet
Count Naffau's *Foot*
   Lieutenant Robert Throckmorton
   Enfign Daniel Fefchens
Earl of Gallwav's *Foot*
   Lieutenant William Garnet
          Francis Piniero
Lieutenant General Hamilton's *Foot*
   Captain Charles Beithe
   Enfign John Starck
Brigadier General Douglas's *Foot*
   Captain Lieutenant John Mackinnon
   Lieutenant John Bail
   Enfign Ifaac Bickerftaff
Sir James Wood's *Foot*
   Lieutenant Richard Symes
         Invalids
   Captain Lewis Gwyn
          Richard Fitz Gerald
   Enfign William Fothot
Independent Companies of the Caftles in
         North-Britain
   Lieutenant William Campbell
Lord Molefworth's *Dragoons*
   Lieut. Colonel Michael de la Bene
   Lieutenant Rigby Molyneux
   Cornet Andrew Bruce
Colonel William Stanhope's *Dragoons*
   Captain Lieut. Marmaduke Taylor
   Cornet Chriftopher Conron
   Surgeon John Hepburn
Sir Charles Hotham's *Dragoons*
   Surgeon Thomas Bates
Sir Robert Rich's *late* Croft's *Dragoons*
   Cornet Charles Stokes
Brigadier General Newton's *Dragoons*
   Cornet Samuel Lowe

                  Brigadier

Brigadier General Ferrers's *Foot.*
 Surgeon Richard Williams
Colonel Maurice Naffau's *Foot.*
 Captain Charles *Lord* Elphinftone
Brigadier General Pocock's *Foot*
 Enfign Ofborn Sidney Wandesford
  Thomas Appiiece
Colonel Hales's *Foot*
 Lieutenant Bury Irwin
Major General Armftrong's *Foot*
 Lieutenant Thomas Griffith
 Enfign Francis Martin
 Adjutant Nathaniel Jackfon
 Surgeon John Middleton
Brigadier General Dubourgay's *Foot*
 Lieut. Gen. David Montolieu, *Baron*
  de St. Hippolite, *as Colonel*
 Lieutenant Thomas Williams
 Enfign Thomas Landey
Brigadier General Pocock's *Foot*
 Captain Elias Brevet
 Enfign Benjamin Wellington
Sir James Wood's *Foot*
 Captain Solomon Defbrifay
  James Bolton
Colonel Groves's *Foot*
 Captain Thomas Webb
Lieutenant General Pearfe's *Foot*
 Quarter Mafter William Ranfon
Lieutenant General Gore's *Dragoons*
 Quarter Mafter James St Amour
Major General Campbell's *Dragoons*
 Cornet Gilbert Pungle
 Quarter Mafter Thomas Lewis
Earl of Stair's *Dragoons*
 Quarter Mafter George Bieton
  George Montgomery
Lieutenant General Evans's *Dragoons*
 Cornet John Lockhart
  John Douglas
Lieutenant General Kerr's *Dragoons*
 Captain George Harrifon
 Quarter Mafter Gerard Bouhier
Lieutenant General Churchill's *Dragoons*
 Captain Robert Napier
 Cornet John Herbert
 Quarter Mafter Freak Duke
Lieutenant General Kirke's *Foot*
 Enfign Robert Hooley
Lieutenant General Tatton's *Foot*
 Enfign John Lambert
Lord Cadogan's *Foot*
 Lieutenant Charles Vachell

Lord Tyrawley's *Foot*
 Lieutenant William Rofs
Lieutenant General Grove's *Foot*
 Enfign Richard Roberts
Lieutenant General Whetham's *Foot*
 Lieutenant John Whitlaw
 Enfign Jofeph Townfend
Lord Mark Kerr's *Foot*
 Enfign John Wind
Earl De Loraine's *Foot*
 Enfign Thomas Dalyell
Lieutenant General Sabine's *Foot*
 Captain Peter Petit
Lieutenant General Tyrrell's *Foot*
 Lieutenant Peter Temple
Brigadier General Kane's *Foot*
 Captain Richard Le Geyt
Colonel Gooch's *Foot* ra 29 Dec. 1739
 Lieutenant Colonel William Merrick
 Major Edward Clarke

Captain -	Richard Riggs William Fitzhugh Peter Dumas Charles Robinfon Herbert Palmer Jofeph De Mellis
Lieutenant -	Thomas Dundas William Cofby Richard Parker William Foye Gilbert Livingftone John Moody Walter Chaloner
Enfign -	Mark Carr Edward Grove Charles Irwin

Regiments, &c diffbanded **1746**
 Doctor Alexander Sandilands, *as*
  Phyfician to the Hofpital in Flanders
Duke of Bedford's *Foot* 1745
 Captain Mufgrave Brifcoe, C F.
Duke of Montagu's *Ordnance* 1745
 Ma. Ch. Ottway, *as Ca of M.*
 Lt. Wm Hull, *as* 1ft *Lt. of Mar.*
  John Gibfon, *as 2d ds.*
Earl of Cholmondeley's *Foot* 1745
 Lt. Col. Vifc. Malpas, *as C. of F.*
 Vifc. Harcourt. *F. ve.* Nov. 13, 1745
 Captain George Davis. *as Enfig.*
Lord Gower's *Foot* ra Oct. 19, 1745
 Lieutenant Walter Chetwynd
Ld Edgcumbe's *F ra.* Dec. 3, 1745
 Mr. Robert Mitford *as C of F.*
         2d

Troops of Guards, &c.

3d Troop of Horfe Guards red. 1746
Juft. Mac Carty, 1ft L. & L. C.
W. Bellenden, 2d Lt. & Lt. C

Philip Browne ⎫ Ex. & Capt
George Phillips ⎭

William Raftall ⎫ Brig & Lt.
Charles Benbow ⎭

John Arnold, Sub Brig & Corn
4th T. of H. G. red. Dec. 24 1746

Clem. Hilgrove ⎫
Robert Auften ⎬ Ex & Capt.
Francis Martin ⎭

John Hopkins ⎫ Brig & Lt.
W. Rob. Adam ⎭

John Bateman ⎫ Sub B. & Cor
Robert Keyte ⎭

C. Hamilton, Adjutant
Edward Darell, Chaplain
See Indepene Comp in North Britain.
Capt Sr Duncan Campbell, Bt.
18 Independ. Comp in North Britain
Capt Patrick Grant, a L. of Foot
Staff-Off. la under L Gl S. Cian
Ja. Abercromby, Com of Maj

Regiments &c. Difbanded and Reduced in 1748 and 1749.

H. R. H the Duke's Drag. red. 1748.
Major James Otway
Captain James Wilkinfon
Lieutenant Nicholas Kirk

Cornet ⎰ John Skitt
⎱ John Palmer

Q. Maf. ⎧ Jonathan Power Gilpin
⎨ Henry Evans
⎪ Henry Addifon
⎩ William Fofter

Adjutant Charles Naylor
Colonel Batereau's Foot broke 1748

Captain ⎧ William Supple
⎨ Bladen Swincy
⎪ John Faire
⎩ George Maxwell

1ft Lieut. ⎧ Robert Spooge
⎨ William Parfons
⎪ Francis Manning
⎪ Richard Grefham
⎩ John Creighton

2d Lieut. ⎰ John Galland
⎱ Michael Bruce

Enfign ⎧ Edward Johnfton
⎨ Allan Jeffryes
⎪ Edmund Turner
⎩ Christopher Woodward

Adjutant Gilbert Tracey
Surgeon Joshua Pilot
Earl of Loudoun's Foot broke 1747-8
Major William Mac Kenzie

Captain ⎧ Edward Brown
⎨ Lord Charles Gordon
⎩ Æneas Mackirtofh

Lieutenant ⎧ Paul Macpherfon
⎨ John Campbell
⎩ Dougall Stewart

Lieutenant ⎰ James Frafer
⎱ Colin Campbell

Enfign ⎰ Robert Grant
⎱ John Benfon

Adjutant Ludowick Grant
Quarter Mafter John Campbell
Lieut. Gen. Churchill's 1ft Marines
Lieut. Col. Nathaniel Mitchell

Captain ⎰ James Carre
⎱ George Buckley

Captain Lt. Richard Phillips

1ft Lieut. ⎧ Alexander Hatfield
⎨ William Tudor
⎩ Hugh Adam

2d Lieut. ⎧ Richard Leigh
⎨ George Coventry
⎪ Charles Johnfton
⎪ David Jones
⎨ Alexander Gordon
⎪ Richard Wadge
⎪ William Alicocke
⎪ John Wyfe
⎩ Mortimer Timpfon

Quarter Mafter Joseph Harris
Surgeon Edward Sabin
Colonel Frafer's 2 Marines

Captain ⎧ George Gibfon
⎨ Robert Foye
⎪ Richard Egan
⎩ Ralph Bendyfhe

1ft Lieut ⎰ John Kirvington
⎱ James Greer

2d Lieut. John Hering
Adjutant Thomas Bennett
Col. Hamerton's Marines
Major Charles Durand

Captain ⎰ John Foulkes
⎱ Alexander Cumming

Corman

Captain	{	Bold Burton
		Ashton Bettles
		Richard Parker
1 Lieut	{	Solomon Sperque
		J. Hen. Milhauet
2 Lieut	{	Hugh Meeke
		Mich. Greenhough
		Herb. Pen ington
		John Sutherland
		Hugh Meredith
		John Bridger
		Joseph Randell
		John Bristol

Adjutant Stephen Browne
Quarter Mr. John Bacon
Surgeon Joseph Parker

Reg. Torrington's 4 *Maons*
Lt. Gen. John Peter Audibert
as *Colonel*
Lt. Col. Boteler Hutchinson

Captain	{	Robert White
		William Roberts
1ft Lieut	{	Henry Moors
		Henry Newton
		Daniel Richardson
		William Werden
		James Donnellan
2d Lieut	{	Thomas Moncrieff
		Geo. L. / Selboun
		Rowland Leffever
		John Greenhaugh
		William Roberts
		John Edwards
		Richard Thompson
		George Mylles
		Cæsar Praten

Quarter Mastr. Peter McLachlan
Lieut. Gen. Cochran's 5 *Maons*
Lt. Col. Charles William Peace

Captain	{	John Bache
		Sir R. Abercromby Bart.
		Sir Pat. Murray Bt.
1ft Lieut	{	Wm Convngham
		John Hay
		Gaston Bernardon
		George Somerville
		William Brien
2d Lieut	{	James Cleland
		John Campbell
		Toomes Balfour

Y

2d Lieut	{	James Stewart
		William North
Surgeon		John Usher

Lieut. Col. Lafore 16 *Maons*
Major Sir Charlton Leighton Bt.

Captain	{	William Hare
		John Bolton
		Goodwin Morton
		Sir J. Arbot, Bt.
1ft Lieut	{	Hector Vaughan
		John Gubbase
2d Lieut	{	Lewis Boundenere
		Howell Lloyd

Surgeon William Hunter
Lt. Col. Cornelius Perry *Maons*

Captain	{	Thomas Moore
		Benjamin Tanaker
		Abraham Clerk

Capt. Lt. George Dick

1ft Lieut	{	John Oock
		David Boos
2d Lieut	{	James Bardolph
		William Selwyn

Surgeon Matthew Bevan
Quarter Mastr. Joseph Shunter
Col. Jordan's 8 *Maons* 1748
Lt. Gen. Sir J. Bruce Hope, Bt.
as *Colonel*
Lt. Col. James Cunningham

Captain	{	Thomas Newton
		George Byron

Capt. Lt. William Bulkley

1ft Lieut	{	Lancelot Simpson
		Hugh Rofe
		James Feeves
2d Lieut	{	David Lauderdale
		John Cofley
		William Hart
		William Courtenay
		James Pope

M. G. Powlett's 9 *Mar brok* 1748
Major Earl of Glencairn

Captain	{	Daniel Robertson
		John Gordon
		William Lawrence
1ft Lieut	{	Thomas Bernard
		Samuel Wilson
		Gerard Daffgn
		William Yalden
		John King
2d Lieut	{	George Wright
		John Douglas

2d Lieut.

2d Lt. { Charles Dundas / Pierce Dent / Henry London / Nathaniel French

Qu. Master John Dodd

Surgeon Nicholas Debat

S.. Agnew's 10 Ma.. b.. 1748

Col Sir Rd Lyttelton, .. Captain.

Captain { John C..on / Arthur Kennedy

1st Lt { Edward John Lyte / Edward Peers / John Hughes

2d Lt { John Cottingham / George Cole / Joseph Dufent / Abraham Brockett / Nicholas Dunbar / Benjamin Pearce / William Laing

L. Gen. St. Clair's add. Comps

Lieut. { James Buchanan / Hugh Forbes

Ensign { George Leith / James Grady / John Tash / Joan Mackay

Qu. Master Benjamin Moodie

Earl of Panmure's add. Comps.

Captain John Bowling

Ensign William Henson

Qu. Master William Grant

Lieu. Gen. Bragg's add. Comps.

Lieutenant Arthur Bragg

Colonel Lee's additional Comps.

Captain David Drummond

Lieut. { Edw Nightingale / Samuel Dash

Ensign John Archer

Colonel Conway's addit Comps.

Ensign Thomas Daniel

L. Gl. Tho. Howard's odd Comps.

Lieutenant Thomas Wayne

Add Comps. of K's own R. 4 Ft.

Lieutenant Thomas Schaak

Ensign John Smith

Add Comps. of K's own Rt of Ft.

Captain Richard Knight

Colonel Bocland's addit. Comps.

Lieutenant David Melville

Ensign Thomas Thompson

Lt. Gen. Skelton's addit. Comps.

Captain Edward Fuller

Captain Mathew Wright

Lt Geo Beauclerck's odd Comps

Lieut. Fran. Wm Shepard

Ensign Francis Houston

Lt Geo Sackville's odd Comp.-

L. William Robinson

Addit Comps North Brit Fus.

Cap.. Campbell Edmonstone

2d Lieut John Lindsay

Addit Comps Welsh Fusi Huske's

Captain Thomas Davis

1st Lieut. John Carter

2d L.. Henry Eyre

Lt Gen Beauclerck's odd Comps.

Captain { John Fleming / George Symes

Lieut. William Marshall

Ensign { Thomas Roche / Joseph Green

Col Leighton's addit Comps.

Ensign Henry Harrison

Lt Gen. Johnson's add Comps.

Captain Eatton Otway

Ensign John Wood

M Gl. Cholmondeley's add Comps.

Ensign { Charles Oates / William Biddolph

Maj. Gl Fleming's add. Comps.

Captain Morris Goulstone

Ensign George Bowes

Colonel Dejean's addit. Comps.

Captain Edward Goddard

Lieutenant Marshall Davis

Royal Rt of Dr. L Gl. Hawley's

Cor en Sec. { Hen. DuVernet / John Johnson / Thomas Gibson / Fran Johnson as Lt. of Foot. / Fran Rainsford

Royal Reg of North Brit Drag.

Cor. en Sec James Campbell

King's own Reg. of Dragoons
Lieutenant General Bland's

Cor en Sec. { William Real / William Wade / Mark Wallis

Sr Robert Rich's Dragoons

Cor. en Sec. Hen Levingstone

Earl of Rothes's Dragoons

Cor. en Sec. { Arch Armstrong / Kean O Hara

Cor.

Cor. en Sec. { Herbert Leighton / George Lindsay / Charles Fluery

Queen's Dragoons, Sir J Cope's

Cor. en Sec. { David Gardiner / Wm Billinge

Lt. Gen. St George's Dragoons

Adjutant Joseph Pendred

Lt. Gen Hampton's Foot

Ensign { John Kelly / Cæsar D'Auvergne / Tho Armstrong / John Leje

Brig Gen Kirkbell's Foot

Ensign { Robert Lindsay / John Poole / John Armstrong

Qu. Master John Fitz-Gerald

Lieutenant Gen Hamson's Foot

Qu. Mast. Henry Bourne

Colonel Munron's Foot

Qu. Master John Lacrousene

Hospital in the Low Countries

James Bringe, Comptroller

John Clephane, Physician

Geo Lawman, Master Surg.

Hospital in North Britain

James Welsh, Surgeon

Staff-Officers in Low Countries

David Cooper, Even Master

Comm... of the Marines

John Arnott, Compiss. Gen

John C... Dep Commissary.

John Scfie, ditto

Charles Hay, ditto

John Pannon, ditto

Col Lt Gl Ja Oglethorpe's Ft.

Lt. Gen. Ja. Oglethorpe or Col

Captain George Dunbar

Lieut. { John Werry's / Paul Moreau / John Mackintosh / Lewis Jones

Ensign { John Stewart / Noble Jones / Thomas Tragge

Qu. Master Patrick Houston

Chaplain David Duval

Surgeon Charles Rolland

Ld John Murray's adit. Corps.

Captain Dougall Campbell

Lieut. { James Campbell / Charles Liliot

Ensign { Patrick Campbell / Peter Grant / Duncan Connbell / Charles Stephens

Earl of Loudoun's a late Co.

Captain { John Sutherland / George Leonard

Lieutenant Daniel M'Neill

Ensign George Monro

Indp. Comps. at South Carolina

Captain Paschal Nelson

Lieut. { Wm Livingstone / James M'Lean / Thomas Lloyd / James Cowley

Major General Fowke's Foot

Qu Master Thomas Major

Lieut. Gen. Haigrave's Foot.

Qu. Mas J. Corgan Chillcott

Lord Tyrawley's Foot

Qu. Mes. John Bourman

Lieut. Gen. Warren's Foot.

Qu. Mes. William Loten

Colonel Kennedy's Foot.

Qu. Mes. Thomas Campbell

Lieutenant General Bragg's Foot.

Qu. Mes Charles Stewart

Lieutenant General Dalzen Foot.

Qu. Mes Crome Outen

Stof. Officer of the late Corps at Loudlingen

Mast. Surgeon { Cherington

Col and Soldier Trothbeck 18.

Captain { George Lewis / Edward Webster / James Birnie / John Winllow / Richard Gadley

Lieut. { John Steele / Edward Powell / William Pass / James Harvey / Charles Proctor / William Cordiner / John Pinkin / James Clark / Charles Ash / ... / Bradders ... / William Harvard / ... Blockholmes

Ensign - { James Hamilton / Josiah Crosby / Richard Abbott

Quarter Master   Joseph Couc

Surgeon   Thomas Wood

Sir William Pepperrell's Foot.

Captain Charles Foyle.

Captain - { David Wooster / Richard Borough / James Vuletres

Lieutenant { John Chamber / William Stewart / Charles Innis / Robert Elliott / Edmond Dwight / Joel Whittemore / Peter Staple / James Grant / Nathaniel Whiting / William Bourne

Ensign - - { William Nelson / Joshua Winslow

Colonel Trelawny's Foot.

Surgeon Robert Cocke

---

12 Ind p Comps from the East Indies.

Captain - { Patrick Lyon / James Dalrymple / John Ramsay / Archibald Grant / Nicholas Price

1st Lieutenant { Lauchl M'Pherson / Donald Campbell / Mathew Feller

2d Lieutenant { Edward Jacob / William Lowes / Robert Duncannon / Peter Gwibal / John Speed / Jasper Saunders / Joseph Cheesbrough / Hugh Fraier / John Grant

Surgeon - { William Stukeley / John Hammond / John Raworth / James Brodie

Hosp. for the late British Forces in Spain. Francis Arbouin, as Director

---

Staff Officers of the late Garrison at Minorca.

Secretaries to the Gov. { Charles Lechmere / Charles Williams

Captain of the Ports   Robert Frampton

Fort St. PHILIP.

Lieutenant Governor   Mordaunt Crocherode

Late Fiftieth Regiment of Foot		Late Fifty-first Regiment of Foot	
Major Gen.	Wm. Shirley, as Col	Major Gen	Sir W. Pepperrell, Col.
Lieut. Colonel	John Littlehales	Major -	Charles Craven
Major -	James Kinneir		
Captain -	{ David Paton / John Vickers / Benjamin Barber / Richard Hunchman / Robert Armstrong	Captain -	{ George Douglas / William Pager / William Williams / Andrew Watkins
Capt. Lieut.	John Cader	Lieutenant -	{ Daniel Tilton / Nathaniel Williams / Richard Pell / Benjamin White / John Cooling
Lieutenant -	{ Thomas Irwin / George Gahan / Joseph Goldthwaite		
Ensign - -	{ Osbourne West / William Coker	Ensign - -	{ Henry Isaac Wendell / James Wedderburn
Chaplain	Philip Lemens	Chaplain -	Jeremiah Watkins
Surgeon -	John Cce		

Allowances

...ances to the Officers and private Gentlemen of the two Troops of H. Guards, and Regiment of Horse, reduced 1746

	l.	s	d			l.	s	d
...oop of H Guards, exclusive of				Brig & Lt. Robert Keyte	73	0	0
· Half Pay	l.	s	d	Brig & Lt. { W. Raftall	73	0	0
& L C Jus. M'Carty	173	7	6	{ Ch Benbow	73	0	0
..L C W. Bel.enden	173	7	6	Sub Br, & Cor. J Arnold	45	12	6
... { Philip Browne	118	12	6	Adjutant Charles Benbow	91	5	0
{ George Phillips	118	12	6	Trump. Andrew Thomas	45	12	6

	l.	s	d		l.	s	d
..fourth Troop				Sub. Brig. Robert Keyte	45	12	0
..m. Hilgrove	118	12	6	Charles Hamilton	91	5	0
...ert Auftin	118	12	6	Adjutant Charles Hamilton	27	7	6
...rcis Martin	118	12	6	Chaplain Edward Darell	30	8	4
Brig. John Hopkins	73	0	0	Trump. Daniel Hopkins	45	12	6
Wm. Robt. Adair	73	0	0	*The King's own Regiment of Horse.*			
Sub. Brig. John Bateman	45	12	6	Lieutenant Thomas Wallis 164	5	0	

Private Gentlemen 3d and 4th Troops on the Allowance of 10l per An. each.

George Darbyshire	Thomas Long	Alex. Farquharson
J. Sweet	John Hering	Stephen Villerett
J Lane	George Weinman	Isaac Lickbarrow
James Ray	Andrew Milne	Lodovic Loddiges
Joseph Fairfax	John Bull	Robert Cope

Superan. Gentlemen of the 4 Tr. H Guards, at 10l 12s 11d. per An each.

Robert Hedley	John Milfan	John Finley
Arthur Alcock	Charles Crouch	John French
William Spence	Thomas Bourne	Samuel Graham
James Per...	Francis Burrit	Thomas Groves
Thomas I....	....Turner	John Hinckley
John Yea..	George Tabener	John Horbins
Richard ...tree	Joseph Slone	William Humphreys
John Noffter	Donald M'Key	William King
Peter Bolton	Walter M'Carter	Peter Brown
John Ram.r	James Rachen	Robert Ormby
John W.....	B.sf Corider	Robert Roome
Daniel P..d	Thomas Wycombe	Lionel Sedier
John French	Jonathan Faton	Thomas Robinson
John Turner	William Pane	Alexander W...
Francis Par.	James Berne	Daniel Farnell
Richard E....	John Teller	Alexander M'Donald
John Arched	John Jones	John Kinkhead
John Burd.	Alexander Cathcart	Christopher Common
John Betley	....	George Pinckot
William Bonif.d	Mathew Harrifon	Roderick M'Kenzie
William C......	Green Camp	John Farian
John G.ham	William Pile	Charles Kerr
Thomas Galloway	David Corb.n	John Lumley
Edward Cheefe	C.C.......	Thomas Burgoyne
Abraham F.....	....	James King
Henry C.............	Th............en	....let Clarke
Francis C..	....	Edward Fothergill
John C........	William ....ne	George Frazard
Mark Pawlett	.... Timmons	Joseph Lecent
John Hofley	.....E. Ibs	Thomas Unock
John Delo	....rB......	William M'Ken.e

At TICONDEROGA. 8 July

Forty-Second REGIMENT of Foot.
Major, Duncan Campbell
Captain Lieutenant, John Campbell
Lieut. { George Farquarfon
{ Hugh M'Pherfon
{ William Baillie
{ John Sutherland
Enfign { Patrick Stuart
{ George Rattray
44 F. Enfign William Frafer
46 F. Lieut Col. Samuel Bearer
Captain { George Needham
{ Edward Wynne
Lieut. { Jacob Laulhé
{ Arthur Lloyd
Enfign { George Crofton
{ Thomas Carbonell
55 F. Colonel George Aug. Vif Howe
Lieut. Col. John Donaldson

Major Thomas Proby
Capt. Lieut. James Murray
Lieutenant George Stuart
60 F. Major John Rutherfurd
Capt. Lieut. Charles Forbes
Lieut. { William Horel
{ Michael Davi
Engineer Mathew Clerk

LOUISBURGH 2
1st (or Royal) REGIMENT of
Lieut. { James Ferton
{ Jofiah How
15 F. Lieut. { Coin Campbel
{ Henry Niche
17 F Captain Wm E of Dundonall
48 F. Enfign Godfrey Roe
8 F Captain Charles Bailie
Lieut. { John Cuthbert
{ John Frafer
{ John Murray

ADDITIONS, &c. since PRINTING.

2 D.	Cornet John M'Dowall	5 Aug. 1758	V.ce. Heron
3 D.	Cornet Huntington Tilden	24 do.	v. Paroi
4 D.	Adjutant Ralph Dundas	do	v. Pov'
7 D.	Lieutenant Samuel Barley	5 do.	v. Manhead
	Cornet John Le Marchand	do	v. Barley
	Adjutant Philip Perry	do	v. Marchand
11 D.	Captain William Lord New battle	24 do.	v. Lindefay
1 F. G	Captain Lieutenant Arthur Graham	do	v. Carleton
8 F.	Lieut Colorel John Mompesson	do.	v. La Fasfille
32 F.	Lieutenant George Swiney	ao.	v Horfley
	Enfign F Schaw	do.	v. Swiney
38 F.	Captain William Adlam	do.	v Staa
	Captain Lieut. Wilson Anderson	do.	v Adlam
	Lieutenant John Kinkead	do.	v. Anderfon
	Enfign Hugh Magenis	do.	v Kinkead
	Adjutant Gilbert Hillock	do.	v. Magenis
50 F.	Lieut. Colonel William Wilkinfon	do.	v. Monckton
54 F.	Lieutenant Henry Harrison	do.	v. Drummond
	Enfign George Hay	do.	v. Harrison
	Quarter-Mufter Fotherg'll	do.	v. Drummond
57 F.	Captain Ch. Kell. County	do.	v. C is
63 F.	Chaplain Richard Kendall	do.	
64 F.	Chaplain Robert Bell	5 do	
66 F.	Colonel John La Fafille	24 do	v. fasfled
69 F.	Enfign Hawker	do.	v. barrer
72 F.	Lieut. Colonel Cur Carleton	do.	v. Weiners

S U C-

UCCESSION

OF

COLONELS,

TO

HIS MAJESTY'S LAND FORCES,
with Dates, Uniforms, &c. 1758.

HORSE-GUARDS.

1 *Red faced Blue, red Farn.* Britain.
G D. of Albemarle 9 *July* 1660
    C. E. of Macclesfield 60
Ja D. of Monmouth 30 *June* 1666
Christ D of Albemarle 29 *Nov* 79
Ls E Feversham 1 *Aug.* 85
Rd. E. Scarborough 2 *Apr.* 89
Arn. E Albemarle, 9 *Mar.* 98-9
H D. Portland 26 *July* 1710
J. E. of Ashburnham 7 *July* 13
J. D. Montagu 10 *Mar* 14-15
H. Ld Herbert 20 *Sept.* 21
J. E. of Westmoreland 4 *July* 33
J. D. Montagu 21 *June* 1737
J. Ld. De Lawarr 30 *Aug.* 37

2 *Troop, Red f. Blue, Blue F.* B
Sir Philip Howard 23 *Nov.* 1659
G.D. of Northumberland 11 *Feb.* 84-5
Ja. D. Ormond 18 *Apr.* 89
G. D. Northumberland 4 *Ja.* 1714-15
Alg. E. of Hertford 8 *Feb.* 13
C D Marlborough 6 *May* 40
Cha. Ld. Cadogan 25 *Apr* 1743

GR. GUARDS.

1 *Red f. Blue, Blue Furn* B at
H. E of Cholmondeley 4 *Oct* 1692
Rd. V. Lumley 8 *Feb.* 1714-15
J E of Westmorland 11 *Dec* 17
R. Rich, Bart 7 *Aug.* 33
C. Hotham, Bart. 13 *May* 35

Ja. Dormer 10 *Feb.* 37-8
Rd. V. Cobham 25 *Dec* 42
Rd. Onslow 25 *Apr.* 45

2 *Red f. Blue, Red Furniture.*
W. Ld. Forbes 12 *May* 1702
J. E. of Craufurd 4 *May* 1704
H E. Marshal 5 *Jan* 13-14
H E Delorane (*removed*) 1 *June* 15
G. Ld Forrester 17 *July* 17
H. Berkeley 21 *Apr.* 19
Fr. E. of Effingham 21 *June* 37
J. E of Craufurd 25 *Dec.* 40
Ja. Ld. Tyrawly 1 *Apr.* 43
J. E. Rothes 25 *Apr.* 45
W. E of Harrington 5 *June* 45

ROYAL HORSE-GUARDS.

Blue faced Red, Red Furniture Br.
Aubrey E. of Oxford 1661
Ja D. of Berwick 4 *Feb.* 87-8
Ja. D. of Hamilton 20 *Nov.* 88
Aubrey E. of Oxford 31 *Dec.* 88
G D Northumberland 13 *Mar.* 1702-3
Rd E. Rivers 4 *Jan.* 11-12
C. E Peterborough 19 *Aug.* 12
J D of Argyll 13 *June* 15
C Marq of Winchester 8 *Mar* 16-17
J. D of Argyll 6 *Aug* 33
Alg E. of Hertford 6 *May* 40
J D of Argyll 24 *Feb* 41-2
Alg D. of Somerset 10 *Mar.* 41-2
C. D. of Richmond 13 *Feb.* 49-50
                    Sir

Sir John Ligonier	27 *Jan.* 53
J. Ms. of Granby	13 *May* 58

1 HORSE, *Red faced Blue, lapelled, pale blue Furniture*, Ireland.

Ja. D. of Hamilton	28 *July* 1685
C. E. of Selkirk	20 *Nov.* 88
C Godfrey	31 *Dec* 88
F. Langstone	7 *Mar.* 92-3
G. Joceline	20 *Oct.* 13
Sherrington Davenport	9 *Feb* 15
O. Wynne,	6 *July* 19
T Pierce	27 *Sp.* 32
Ja. Ld Tyrawly	26 *Aug* 39
J. Brown	1 *Apr.* 43

2 *Red faced full Green, lapelled, full green Furniture*, Ireland.

C. D. of Shrewsbury	29 *July* 1685
Marmaduke Ld Langdale	22 *Ja.* 86-7
R. Hamilton	15 *Feb.* 86-7
J. Coy	31 *Dec.* 88
C. Butler, E Arran	1 *July* 97
W. E. of Cadogan	2 *Mar.* 2-3
G. Kellum	22 *Dec.* 12
R. Napier	27 *May* 17
Clement Neville	6 *May* 40
Rd. Vt. Cobham	5 *Aug* 44
T. Wentworth	20 *June* 15
T. Bligh	22 *Dec.* 47

3 *Red faced pale Y. lap. pale y. Fur.* Ir.

Rd. Ld. Lumley	31 *July* 1685
Sir John Talbot	29 *Jan.* 86-7
Vt. Hewet	31 *Dec* 88
R. Beverley	30 *Dec.* 89
Hugh Wyndham	31 *Jan.* 91-2
Fr. Palmes	1 *Oct.* 1706
Leigh Backwell	2 *Apr.* 12
Rd Waring	15 *Feb.* 14-15
Rd Visc. Shannon	17 *June* 21
G. Maccartney	9 *Mar.* 26-7
H. E. of Deloraine	9 *July* 30
R. Rich, Bart.	1 *Jan.* 30-1
C. Ld Cathcart	7 *Aug.* 33
Phineas Bowles	20 *Dec.* 40
Ja. Cholmondeley	1 *Nov.* 49
Ld G. Sackville	18 *Jan.* 49-50
Ls. Dejean	5 *Apr.* 57

4 *Red faced Black, lap. Buff-co. F* Ir.

W. Ld Cavendish	31 *Dec* 1688
Mainhard D. of Schomberg	10 *Ap* 90

C. Ms. of Harwich his S.	27 *Ja* 10
C. Sybourg	12 *Oct*
Sir John Ligonier	18 *July*
Sir J. Mordaunt	24 *July*
H de Grangues	1 *Nov*
H. Conway	8 *July*

1 KING's DRAGOON GUAR
***Red f. Blue, red Furniture,* Br**

Sir J. Lanier	6 *June* 1685
H Lumley	10 *Aug*
Rd. V. Irwin	13 *Dec*
Rd. V. Cobham	10 *Ap.*
H. E. Pembroke	22 *Jul*
Sir Ph Honywood	18 *Ap*
Humph. Bland	8 *Jul*

2 QUEEN's *ditto, Red, f. Buff col. half Lapel., Buff* F. B.

H E. Peterborough	20 *June* 1685
Ed. Villiers,	31 *Dec.* 1688
Rd. Leveson	19 *Jan* 1693-4
Dan. Harvey	25 *Mar.* 99
John Bland	1 *Jan.* 11-12
T. Pitt, E. Londonderry	9 *Fel.* 14-15
J D Argyil	26 *Aug.* 26
W. Evans	6 *Aug* 33
J D. Montagu	6 *May* 40
Sir John Ligonier	24 *July* 49
Hon. W. Herbert	27 *Jan.* 53
Ld G. Sackville	5 *Apr* 57

3 Dr. G. *Red. f. White, half Lapel., wb Fur.* Brit.

T. E Plymouth	15 *July* 1685
Sir J. Fenwick	6 *Nov* 87
Rd. E. Rivers	31 *Dec.* 88
J. Ld Berkeley of Stratton	23 *Ja.* 91-2
Cornelius Wood	1 *Dec* 93
T. Visc Windsor	13 *May* 1712
G. Wade	19 *Mar.* 16-17
C. Howard, Kt B.	15 *Mar.* 47-8

1. ROYAL DRAGOONS.
***Red, faced Blue, red Furn.* Brit.**

J Ld Churchill	19 *Nov.* 1683
Ed. V. Cornbury	1 *Aug* 85
R. Clifford	24 *Nov* 88
Ed. V. Cornbury	31 *Dec.* 88
Ant Hayford	1 *July* 89
Ed. Mathews	24 *Oct.* 94
T Ld Raby E. Strafford	30 *May* 97

Rd. Vis.

Richard Vt. Cobham 13 *June* 1715
Charles Hotham, Bart. 10 *Apr* 21
Humphry Gore 12 *Jan* 22-3
Charles D. of Marlborough 1 *Sept.* 39
Henry Hawley 12 *May* 40

2 *R. N. B. R. faced Blue, blue* F. B.
Thomas Dalzell 25 *Nov.* 1681
Charles E. Dunmore 6 *Nov.* 85
Thomas Ld Tiviot 31 *Dec.* 88
Ld. John Hay 7 *Apr.* 1704
John E. Stair 24 *Aug.* 1706
David E. Portmore 21 *Apr.* 14
Sir James Campbell 15 *Feb.* 16 17
John E. Stair 28 *May* 45
John E. of Craufurd 22 *May* 47
John E. of Rothes 17 *Jan.* 49-50
John Campbell 29 *Apr.* 52

3 *King's own Regiment, Red, faced light Blue, light blue Furniture* B
Charles D. of Somerset 2 *Aug.* 1685
Alexander Cannon 2 *Aug.* 87
Richard Leveson 31 *Dec.* 88
Thomas Ld Fairfax 20 *Jan* 93-4
William Lloyd 21 *Feb.* 94-5
George Ld Carpenter 31 *Dec.* 1703
Philip Honywood 29 *May* 32
Humphry Bland 18 *Apr.* 43
Ld Tyrawly 8 *July* 52
George E. of Albemarle 8 *Apr.* 55

4 *Red faced Green, Green Furn.* Br.
John V. Fitzharding 17 *July* 1685
Thomas Maxwell 24 *Nov.* 88
John V. Fitzharding 13 *Dec.* 88
Algernon E. of Essex 1 *Sept.* 93
Sir Richard Temple 24 *Apr.* 1710
William Evans 12 *Oct.* 13
Robert Rich, Bart. 13 *May* 35

5 *Royal Irish, Red f. Blue, bl* F. Ir.
James Wynne 25 *Dec.* 1689
Charles Ross 16 *July* 95
Thomas Sydney 8 *Oct.* 1715
Charles Ross 1 *Feb.* 28-9
Owen Wynne 6 *Aug.* 32
Richard V. Molesworth 27 *June* 37

6 *Inniskilling, Red faced full Yellow, full Yellow Furniture,* Britain.
Sir Albert Cunningham 31 *Dec.* 1688
Robert Echlyn 30 *Dec.* 91
John E. of Stair 4 *Mar.* 1714-15
Charles Ld Cadogan 10 *Jan.* 24

John E. of Stair 25 *Apr.* 1743
John E. of Rothes 29 *May* 45
James Cholmondeley 18 *Jan.* 49-50

7 *Queen's, Red faced White, wh.* F.B.
Richard Cunningham 30 *Dec.* 1690
William Ms Lothian 1 *Oct.* 96
Patrick Ld Polwarth 28 *Apr.* 1707
William Kerr 10 *Oct.* 9
John Cope, Kt B. 12 *Aug.* 41

8 *Red faced Yellow, yellow Furn.* Ir.
Henry Cunningham 1 *Feb.* 1692-3
Robert Killigrew 26 *Jan.* 1705-6
John Pepper 15 *Apr.* 07
Phineas Bowles 23 *Mar* 18-19
Richard Munden 19 *Nov.* 22
Robert Rich, Bt 20 *Sept* 25
Charles Cathcart 1 *Jan.* 30-1
Sir Adam Oughton 7 *Aug.* 33
Clement Neville 27 *June* 37
Richard St. George 6 *May* 40
John Waldegrave 22 *Jan* 55

9 *Red faced Buff, Buff-col. Furn.* Ir.
Owen Wynne 22 *July* 1715
James Crofts 6 *July* 19
Richard Vt. Molesworth 29 *May* 32
John Cope 27 *June* 37
John Brown 10 *May* 42
Henry de Grangues 1 *Apr.* 43
George Read 1 *Nov.* 49
John Jorden 2 *Apr.* 56
Philip Honywood 22 *May* 56

10 *Red faced deep Yellow, deep y.* F. B.
Humphry Gore 22 *July* 1715
Charles Churchill 12 *Jan.* 22-3
Richard Visc. Cobham 1 *June* 45
Sir John Mordaunt 1 *Nov.* 49

11 *Red faced Buff, buff col. Furn.* B.
Philip Honywood 22 *July* 1715
Ld Mark Kerr 29 *May* 32
William E. of Ancram 8 *Feb.* 52

12 *Red faced White, white Furn.* Ir.
Phineas Bowles 22 *July* 1715
Phineas Bowles 23 *Mar* 18-19
Alexander Rose 20 *Dec.* 40
Sir Warter Whitshed 14 *June* 43
Thomas Bligh 6 *Apr.* 46
Sir John Mordaunt 22 *Dec.* 47
James Cholmondeley 24 *July* 49
Ld George Sackville 1 *Nov.* 49
John Whitefoord, Bt. 18 *Jan.* 50

Y 13 *R. d*

13 *Red faced light Green, do. Fur.* Ir

Richard Munden	22 *July* 1715
Robert Rich, Ba.t	19 *Nov* 22
William Earl of Harrington	20 *Sept* 25
Henry Hawley	7 *July* 30
Robert Dalway	12 *May* 40
Humphry Bland	9 *Jan* 40-1
James Gardner	18 *Apr.* 43
Francis Ligonier	1 *Oct* 45
Philip Naizon	17 *Feb* 44-5
Sir Ch. Armand Powlet	26 *Jan* 50-51
Henry Conway	25 *Dec* 51
John Moflyn	8 *July* 54

14 *Red faced lemon Colour, do Fur* Ir

James Dormer	22 *July* 1715
Clement Neville	9 *Apr.* 20
Arch.bald Hamilton	27 *June* 37
James Lord Tyrawly	24 *July* 49
Lewis Dejean	27 *Nov.* 52
John Campbell	5 *Apr* 57

1 FOOT-GUARDS, 3 *Battalions* British *Red faced Blue, white Lace, white Lace Shoulder-Strap*

John Ruffel	23 *Nov* 1660
Henry D. Grafton	14 *Dec.* 81
Edward E. Litchfield	30 *Nov* 88
Henry D Grafton	31 *Dec.* 88
Henry E. Romney	16 *Mar.* 88-9
Charles D. Schomberg	27 *Dec.* 91
Henry E. Romney	20 *Nov* 93
John D Marlborough	25 *Apr.* 1704
James D. Ormond	1 *Jan* 11-12
John D. Marlborough	26 *Sept.* 14
William E Cadogan	18 *June* 22
Charles Willes, Kt. B.	26 *Aug.* 26
Wm. D. of Cumberland	18 *Feb.* 41-2
John Visc. Ligonier	3 *Nov.* 57

2 Coldstream, *Red faced Blue, laced, flofh Pockets,* B

George D. Albemarle	26 *Aug.* 1650
William E Craven	6 *Jan.* 69-70
Thomas Talmafh	1 *May* 89
John Ld. Cutts	3 *Oct.* 94
Charles Churchill	25 *Feb.* 1706-7
William Cadogan	11 *Oct.* 14
Richard E. Scarborough	18 *Jan* 22
William D. Cumberland	23 *Apr* 40
Charles D. Marlborough	18 *Feb.* 41-2
William A. E. Albemarle	5 *Oct* 44
James Ld. Tyrawly	8 *Apr.* 55

3 Scotc' *Red faced Blue, white Lace,* B.

George E Linlithgow	23 *Nov* 1660
James Douglas	13 *June* 84
Charles Ramfay	1 *Oct* 91
William Ms. of Lothian	25 *Apr.* 1707
John E Dunmore	10 *Oct* 13
John E. Rothes	29 *Apr.* 52

1 FOOT, *Royal Regiment, 2 Battalions Red faced Blue, Ireland and America.*

Sir John Hepburn	26 *Jan.* 1633
John Hepburn	26 *Aug.* 1636
Ld. James Douglas	1637
George E Dunbarton	21 *Oct* 45
Frederick D Schomberg	31 *Dec* 88
Sir Robert Douglas	5 *Mar.* 90-1
George E Orkney	1 *Jan* 92
James St. Clair	27 *June* 1737

2 Queen's *Royal Regiment, Red, faced Sea-Green,* Ireland.

Henry E Peterborough	30 *Sept* 1661
Andrew E Tiviot	9 *Apr.* 63
Henry Norwood	10 *Oct.* 1664
Charles E. Middleton	15 *May* 68
William E Inchiquin	5 *Mar* 74-5
Sir Palmes Fairborne	10 *Nov.* 80
Piercy Kirke	19 *Apr.* 82
William Selwyn	18 *Dec* 91
Sir Henry Bellafis	28 *June* 1701
David E. Portmore	27 *Feb.* 02-3
Piercy Kirke	19 *Sept.* 10
Thomas Fowke	12 *Aug.* 41
John Fitzwilliam	12 *Nov.* 55

3 Buffs, *Red faced Buff,* Brit.

Robert Sydney	31 *May* 1665
Sir Walter Vane	12 *Aug.* 68
John E Mulgrave	12 *Dec.* 73
Philip E Chefterfield	6 *Nov.* 82
John E. Mulgrave	26 *Jan* 83-4
Sir Theophilus Oglethorpe	25 *Oct* 85
Charles Churchill	31 *Dec* 88
John D. Argyll	24 *Feb* 1706-7
John Selwyn	26 *Feb.* 10-11
Archibald E Forfar	14 *Apr* 13
Charles Wills	5 *Jan.* 15-16
Thomas E Londonderry	26 *Aug.* 26
William Tatton	24 *Nov.* 29
Thomas Howard	27 *Jan.* 37
George Howard	21 *Aug.* 49

4 King's

4 King's own Regiment, Red f Blue, B.
Charles E. Plymouth   13 July 1680
Percy Kirke   27 Nov 80
Charles Trelawny   23 Apr. 82
Sir Charles Osby   11 Dec. 88
Charles Trelawny   12 Feb 84-5
Henry Trelawny   1 Jan. 91-2
William Seymour   12 Feb 1701-2
Henry Berkeley   25 Dec 1717
Charles Ld Cadogan   21 Apr 19
William Barrell   8 Aug 34
Robert Rich   22 Aug 49
Alexander Duroure   12 May 56

5 Red faced Gosling green, B.
John Obrian V. Clare   1674
John Fenwick, Bt.   26 Aug. 75
Henry Wisely   11 Sept. 76
Thomas Monk   10 Dec 80
Thomas Talmash   9 Oct 80
Edward Lloyd   1 May 89
Thomas Fairfax   6 Nov 94
Thomas Pearce   5 Feb. 1703-4
John Cope   15 Dec. 32
Alexander Irwine   27 June 37
Charles Whitefoord   25 Nov 52
Lord George Bentinck   20 Aug 54

6 Red faced deep Yellow, Gib.altar.
Sir Walter Vane   12 Dec 1673
Luke Lillingston   16 Aug 74
Thomas Alley   13 Sept. 77
Sir Henry Belasis   3 Apr. 80
William Babington   28 Sept 89
Geo. Prince HesseDarmstadt   15 Apr. 91
Henry Ms de Rada   1 Feb. 93-4
Ventris Columbine   23 June 95
James Rivers   2 Nov. 1703
William Southwell   6 Feb 05-6
Thomas Harrison   14 June 08
Robert Dormer   7 Mar. 15-16
James Dormer   9 Apr. 20
John Guise   1 Nov. 38

7 Royal English Fusileers, Red faced Blue, Gibraltar.
George Lord Dartmouth   11 June 85
John Lord Churchill   26 Aug. 89
George Earl Orkney   23 Jan 91-2
Edward Fitzpatrick   1 Aug 92
Charles Lord Tyrawly   12 Nov 96
James Lord Tyrawly   29 Jan. 1712-13

William Hargrave   27 Aug. 1739
John Mostyn   26 Jan. 50-1
Lord Robert Bertie   12 Aug 54

8 King's, Red faced Blue, Eng.
Robert Lord Ferrers   19 June 1685
James Duke of Berwick   1 Nov 86
John Beaumont   31 Dec 88
John Richmond Webb   26 Dec 95
Henry Morrison   5 Aug 1715
Sir Charles Hotham   3 Dec 20
John Pocock   21 Apr 21
Charles Lance   8 May 32
Richard O flow   6 June 39
Edward Wolfe   25 Apr. 45

9 Red faced Yellow, Ir.
Henry Cornwall   19 7bre 1685
Oliver Nicholas   20 Nov 83
John Cunningham   31 Dec 83
William Stewart   1 May 89
James Campbell   27 July 1715
Charles Lord Cathcart   15 Feb. 16-17
James Otway   7 Jan. 17-18
Richard Kane   25 Dec. 25
William Hargrave   27 Jan 37
George Read   28 Aug 39
Sir Charles Armand Powlet   1 Nov. 49
John Waldegrave   26 Jan. 50-1
Hon. Joseph Yorke   13 Mar. 55

10 Red faced bright Yellow, Ir.
John Earl of Bath   20 Jan 1685
Sir Charles Carney   8 Dec. 83
John Earl of Bath   31 Dec 88
Sir Beville Granville   29 Oct. 93
Wm Ld North & Grey   15 Jan 1702-3
Henry Grove   23 June 15
Francis Columbine   27 June 37
James Lord Tyrawly   26 Dec 46
Edward Pole   10 Aug. 49

11 Red faced full Green, Jersey
Henry D of Beaufort   20 June 1685
Charles Ms. of Worcester   26 Oct. 85
William Marquis of Powis   8 May 87
Sir John Hanmer   31 Dec. 88
James E. of Stanhope   12 Feb. 1701-2
John Hill   8 May 5
Edward Montague   13 July 15
Stephen Cornwallis   9 Aug. 38
Robinson Sowle   21 May 43

William

William Graham 7 *Feb* 1745-6
Maurice Bocland 1 *Dec.* 47

12 *Red faced Yellow*, Germ.

Henry D. of Norfolk 20 *June* 1685
Edward E. of Litchfield 14 *June* 86
Robert l d Hunsdon 30 *Nov.*
Henry W .a ton 31 *Dec.* 88
Robert B.ewer 1 *Nov.* 89
John Live ay 28 *Sept.* 1702
Richard Fhilips 16 *Mar.* 11-12
Thomas Stanwix 25 *Aug.* 17
Thomas Whetham 22 *Mar.* 24-5
Scipio du Roure 12 *Aug* 41
Henry Skelton 28 *May* 45
Robert Napier 22 *Apr* 57

13 *Red Faced philemot Yellow*, Gibral.

TheophilusE.Huntingdon20*Jan.*1685
Ferdinando Haftings 20 *Nov.* 88
Sir John Jacobs 13 *Mar.* 94-5
JamesE. of Barrymore 15 *Mar.*1701-2
Stanhope Cotton 28 *July* 15
Ld. Mark Kerr 25 *Dec.* 25
John Middleton 29 *May* 32
Harry Pulteney 5 *July* 39

14 *Red faced Buff*, Gibraltar.

Edward Hales, Bt. 22 *June* 1685
William Beveridge 31 *Dec.* 88
John Tidcomb 14 *Nov.* 92
Jafper Clayton 15 *June* 1713
John Price 22 *June* 43
William Herbert 1 *Dec.* 47
Edward Braddock 17 *Feb.* 53
Thomas Fowke 12 *Nov.* 55
Charles Jefferyes 7 *Sept.* 56

15 *Red faced Yellow*, Am.

William Clifton, Bt. 22 *June* 1685
Arthur E 'Torrington 12 *May* 86
Sackville Tufton 12 *Apr.* 87
Sir James Lefley 31 *Dec.* 88
Emanuel How 1 *Nov.* 95
Algernon E. of Hertford 23 *Oct.*1709
Henry Harrifon 8 *Feb.* 14-15
John Jorden 15 *Apr.* 49
Jeffery Amherft 22 *May* 56

16 *Red faced Yellow*, Ir.

Archibald Douglas 9 *Oct.* 1688
Robert Hodges 31 *Dec.* 88
James E. Derby 1 *Aug.* 92

Francis Godfrey 25 *Mar.* 1705
Henry Durell 17 *Feb.* 10-11
Hans Hamilton 23 *June* 13
Richard Vifc. Irwin 11 *July* 15
John Cholmeley 13 *Dec.* 17
Henry E. of Deloraine 7 *Apr.* 24
Roger Handafyd 9 *July* 30

17 *Red faced greyifh White*, Am.

Solomon Richards 27 *Sept.* 1688
Sir George St. George 1 *May* 89
John Courthorpe 1 *Mar.* 94-5
Sir Mathew Bridges 1 *Sept.* 95
Holcroft Blood 26 *Aug* 1703
John Whitman 20 *Aug.* 7
Thomas Ferrers 28 *Sept.* 22
James Tyrrell 7 *Nov.* 22
John Wynyard 31 *Aug* 42
Edward Richbell 14 *Mar.* 52
John Forbes 25 *Feb* 57

18 *Royal* Irifh, *Red faced Blue*, Ir.

Arthur E. of Granard 1 *Apr.* 1683
Arthur Ld Forbes, *his Son*1 *Mar.* 85-6
Sir John Edgeworth 31 *Dec.* 88
Edward E. of Meath 1 *May* 89
Frederick Hamilton 1 *Oct.* 96
Richard Ingoldfby 1 *Apr.* 1705
Richard Stearne 18 *Feb.* 11-12
William Cofby 24 *Dec* 17
Charles Hotham, Bt. 7 *Jan.* 31-2
John Armftrong 13 *May* 35
John Mordaunt 18 *Dec.* 42
John Folliot 22 *Dec.* 47

19 *Red faced yellowifh Green*, Br.

Francis Lutterell 20 *Nov.* 1688
Thomas Erle 1 *Jan.* 90-1
George Freake 23 *Mar.* 1708-9
Richard Sutton 3 *Apr.* 12
George Grove 5 *Aug.* 15
Richard Sutton 27 *Oct.* 29
Hon. Charles Howard 1 *Nov.* 38
Ld. George Beauclerck 15 *Mar.* 47-8

20 *Red faced pale Yellow*, Germ.

Robert Peyton, Bt. 20 *Nov.* 1688
Guftavus Vif. Boyne 1 *June* 89
John Newton 1 *May* 1706
Thomas Meredith 4 *Oct.* 14
William Egerton 7 *July* 19
Francis E. of Effingham 22 *July* 32
Richard St. George 27 *June* 37

Alexander

Alexander Rofe 6 *May* 1740
Thomas Bligh 26 *Dec.* 40
Ld George Sackville 9 *Apr.* 46
Geo.ge Vif. Bury 1 *Nov.* 49
Philip Honywood 8 *Apr.* 55
William Kingfley 22 *May* 56

21 *North Brit. Fuziliers,* R. f. Bl G.b.

Charles E. of Marr 23 *Sept.* 1678
Thomas Buchan 29 *July* 86
Francis Fergus Offarrell 1 *Mar.* 88-9
Robert Macray 13 *Nov.* 95
Archiba'd Row 1 *Jan.* 96-7
John Vt. Mordaunt 25 *Aug* 1704
Sampfon de Lalo 26 *June* 06
John Vt. Mordaunt 4 *Sept.* 09
Thomas Meredith 1 *May* 10
Charles E. of Orrery 8 *Dec.* 10
George Mackartney 12 *July* 16
Sir James Wood 9 *Mar.* 26-7
John Campbell 1 *Nov.* 38
E. of Panmure 29 *Apr.* 52

22 *Red faced pale Buff,* Nova-Scotia.

Henry D. of Norfolk 16 *Mar.* 1688-9
Henry Bellafis, Kt. 28 *Sept.* 89
William Selwyn 28 *June* 1701
Thomas Handafyd 20 *June* 1702
Roger Handafyd 3 *Apr.* 12
William Barrell 25 *Aug.* 30
James St. Clair 30 *Oct.* 34
John Moyle 27 *June* 37
Thomas Paget 15 *Dec.* 38
Richard Offarrell 12 *Aug.* 41
Edward Whitmore 11 *July* 57

23 *Royal Welfh Fuziliers, Red faced Blue,* Germ.

Charles Herbert 12 *May* 1686
Henry Ld Herbert 17 *Mar.* 88-9
Toby Purcell 13 *July* 91
John Morgan, Bt. 20 *Apr.* 92
Robert Ingoldfby 28 *Feb.* 92-3
Jofeph Sabine 1 *Apr.* 1705
Newfham Peers 23 *Nov* 39
John Hufke 28 *July* 43

24 *Red lined white, faced will. Gr.* B.

Edward Dering, Bt. 18 *Mar.* 1688-9
Daniel Dering 27 *Sept.* 89
Samuel Venner 1 *June* 91
Lewis Marq. de Puizar 13 *Mar.* 94-5

William Seymour 1 *Mar.* 1700-1
John E. Marlborough 12 *Feb.* 01-2
William Tatton 25 *Aug.* 04
Gilbert Primrofe 9 *Mar.* 07-8
Thomas Howard 10 *Sept.* 17
Thomas Wentworth 27 *June* 37
Daniel Houghton 21 *June* 45
William E. of Ancram 1 *Dec.* 45
Edward Cornwallis 8 *Feb.* 52

25 *Red faced deep Yellow,* Germ.

David E. of Leven 19 *Mar.* 1688
James Maitland 19 *Mar* 93-4
William Bretton 15 *Apr.* 1711
Richard V. Shannon 27 *Jan.* 14-15
John Middleton 17 *June* 21
John E. of Rothes 29 *May* 32
Francis Ld Sempill 25 *Apr.* 45
John E. of Craufurd 26 *Dec.* 46
William E. of Panmure 1 *Dec.* 47
William E. Home 29 *Apr.* 52

26 *Red faced pale Yellow,* Ir.

James . of Angus 13 *Apr.* 1689
Andrew Monro 1 *Aug.* 92
James Fergufon 25 *Aug.* 93
James Borthwick 24 *Oct.* 1705
John E. of Stair 1 *Jan.* 05-6
George Prefton 24 *Aug.* 06
Philip Anftruther 3 *May* 20

27 Innifkilling, *Red faced Buff,* Am.

Zachariah Tiffin 20 *June* 1689
Thomas Whetham 29 *Aug* 1702
Richard Molefworth 22 *Mar.* 24-5
Archibald Hamilton 29 *May* 32
William Ld Blakeney 27 *June* 37

28 *Red faced bright Yellow,* Am.

John Gibfon, Kt. 16 *Feb.* 1693-4
Sampfon de Lalo 1 *Feb* 1703-4
John Vt. Mordaunt 29 *June* 06
Andrew Windfor 1 *Oct.* 09
William Barrell 27 *Sep.* 15
Nicholas Price 25 *Aug* 30
Philip Bragg 10 *Oct.* 34

29 *Red faced Yellow,* Ireland.

Thomas Farrington 12 *Feb* 1701-2
Ld Mark Keir 7 *Oct.* 12
Henry Defney 25 *Dec.* 25
William A. E. of Albemarle 22 *Nov.* 31
George

George Read 5 *June* 1733
Francis Fuller 28 *Aug* 39
Peregrine Thomas Hopson 6 *June* 48
George Boscawen 4 *Mar* 52

30 *Red faced pale Yellow*, Britain.
Thomas Saunderson 12 *Feb.* 1701-2
Thomas Pownell 15 *Dec.* 04
Charles Willis 13 *Oct.* 05
George Ld Forrester 5 *Jan* 15-16
Thomas Stanwix 17 *July* 17
Andrew Bissett 25 *Aug* 17
Henry de Grangues 24 *Oct.* 42
Charles Frampton 1 *Apr.* 43
John E. of Loudoun 1 *Nov.* 49

31 *Red fared Buff*, Britain.
George Villiers 12 *Feb* 1701-2
Alexander Lutterell 6 *Dec.* 03
Josiah Churchill 1 *Feb.* 05-6
Harry Goring, Bt. 1 *Mar* 10-11
Ld John Kerr 8 *Sept.* 15
Charles Cathcart 13 *Aug.* 28
William Hargrave 1 *Jan.* 30
William Handasyd 27 *June* 37
Ld Henry Beauclerck 25 *Apr* 45
Henry Holmes 8 *May* 49

32 *Red faced White*, B.
Edward Fox 12 *Feb* 1701-2
Jacob Borr 5 *Dec* 04
Charles Dubourgay 26 *June* 23
Thomas Paget 28 *July* 37
Simon Delcury 15 *Dec* 38
John Huske 25 *Dec* 40
John Skelton 27 *Aug* 43
William Douglas 29 *May* 45
Francis Leighton 1 *Dec* 47

33 *Red Laced White*, Britain.
Lt Gen. Stanhope 12 *Feb.* 1701-2
George E. of Huntingdon 12 *Feb.* 01-2
Henry Leigh 04
Robert Duncanson 05
George Wade 9 *Jan.* 05
Henry Hawley 19 *Mar* 16-17
Robert Dalzell 9 *July* 30
John Johnson 7 *Nov.* 39
Ld Charles Hay 20 *Nov.* 53

34 *Red faced bright Yellow* Britain.
Robert Ld Lucas 12 *Feb.* 1701-2
Hans Hamilton 1 *Feb.* 04-5

Thomas Chudleigh 30 *Nov.* 1712
Robert Hayes 18 *Feb.* 22-3
Stephen Cornwallis 8 *Jan.* 31-2
Ld James Cavendish 1 *Nov.* 28
James Cholmondeley 18 *Dec* 42
Henry Conway 24 *July* 49
John Russel 17 *Dec* 51
Thomas Earl of Effingham 2 *Dec.* 54

35 *Red faced Orange*, America.
Arthur E. of Donnegal 28 *June* 1701
Richard Gorges 15 *Apr.* 06
Charles Otway 26 *July* 17

36 *Red faced Green*, Britain.
William Vt. Charlemont 28 *June* 1701
Thomas Allnut 10 *May* 06
Archibald E. of Isla 23 *Mar* 08-9
Henry Desney 23 *Oct.* 10
William Egerton 11 *July* 15
Charles Hotham, Bart. 7 *July* 19
John Pocock 2 *Dec* 20
Charles Lanoe 21 *Apr.* 21
John Moyle 14 *May* 32
Humphry Bland 27 *June* 37
James Fleming 9 *Jan* 40-1
Ld Robert Manners 23 *Mar* 50-1

37 *Red faced Yellow*, Germ
Thomas Meredith 13 *Feb* 1701-2
William Windress 1 *May* 10
John E. of Westmoreland 23 *Aug* 15
Edward V Hinchinbroke 11 *Dec.* 17
Hon. Robert Murray 4 *Aug* 22
Henry Ponsonby 13 *May* 35
Sir Robert Monro 17 *June* 45
Lewis Dejean 9 *Apr* 46
James Stuart 27 *Nov* 52

38 *Red faced Yellow*, Leeward Islands.
Luke Lillingston 13 *Feb* 1701-2
James Jones 2 *June* 08
Francis Alexander 27 *Nov.* 11
Richard Lucas 23 *Sept.* 17
Edward Jones 25 *Dec* 29
Hon. Robert Murray 13 *May* 35
Charles D. of Marlborough 30 *Mar* 38
Robert Dalzell 7 *Nov.* 39
Richard Phillips 13 *May* 49-50
Alexander Durowe 27 *Feb* 50-1
Sir James Lockhart Ross Bt 26 *Mar* 50

39 *Red*

39 Red faced Green, Brit.

Richard Coote	13 Feb 1701-2
Nicholas Sankey	17 Mar. 03
Thomas Ferrers	11 Mar. 19
William Newton	23 Sept. 22
John Cope	10 Nov. 30
Thomas Wentworth	15 Dec 32
John Campbell	27 June 37
Richard Onflow	1 Nov. 38
Robert Dalway	6 Fr w 39
Samuel Whiter Whitfhed	28 Dec 40
Edward Richbell	14 June 43
John Adlercron	14 Mar. 52

40 Red faced Buff, Plantations.

Richard Philips	25 Aug. 1717
Edward Cornwallis	13 Mar. 49-50
Peregrine Thomas Hopton	4 Mar. 52

41 Red faced Blue, Invalids, Britain.

Edmond Fielding	11 Mar 1718-29
Tomkins Wardour	1 Apr. 49
John Parfons	4 Mar. 52

42 or Royal Highland Regt. Red faced Blue, belted Plaid and Hofe, 2 Batt. America.

John E. of Craufurd	25 Oct 1739
Francis Ld Sempill	14 Jan 40 1
Ld John Murray	25 Apr 45

43 Red faced White, Am.

Thomas Fowke	3 Jan. 1740-1
William Graham	12 Aug 41
James Kennedy	7 Feb. 45-6

44 Red faced Yellow, Nova-Scotia.

James Long	7 Jan 1740-1
John Lee	11 Mar. 42-3
Philip Halket, Bart	26 Feb 51
Robert Ellifon	13 Nov. 55
James Abercromby	13 Mar 56

45 Red faced deep Green, Plantations.

Daniel Houghton	11 Jan. 1740-1
Hugh Warburton	22 June 45

46 Red faced Yellow, Am.

John Price	13 Jan 1740-1
Thomas Murray	23 Jan 43

47 Red faced White, Plantations

John Mordaunt	15 Jan 1740-1
Peregrine Lafcelles	13 Mar 42-3

48 Red faced Buff, Nova-Scotia

James Cholmondeley	17 Jan. 1740-1
Ld Harry Beauclerck	14 Mar. 42-3
Francis Ligonier	25 Apr. 45
Henry Conway	6 Apr. 46
George V Torrington	24 July 49
William E. Home	11 Apr 50
Thomas Dunbar	29 Apr. 52
Daniel Webb	11 Nov 55

49 Red faced Full Green, Jamaica.

Edward Trelawney	25 Dec. 1743
George Wulfh	22 Jan. 54

50 Black white Lining, white Lace, Br.

James Abercromby	18 Dec. 1755
Stucholme Hodgion	30 May 56

51 Sea Green, yellow Lace, Germ.

Robert Napier	19 Dec. 1755
Thomas Prudenell	22 Apr. 57

52 Buff, yellow Lace, Ir.

Helworth Lambton	20 Dec. 1755
Edward Sandford	7 June 58

53 Red, yellow Lining, yell. Lace, Gib.

William Whitmore	21 Dec. 1755

54 Popinjay Green, white Lace, Gib.

John Campbell	23 Dec. 1755
John Grey	5 Apr 57

55 Deep Green, yellow Lace, Am.

Charles Perry	25 Dec 1755
George Auguftus Vt.Howe	28 Sept. 57

56 Deep Colour, white Lace, Pink from Britain.

Ld Charles Manners	26 Dec. 1755

57 Lemon Colour, yellow Lace, Gib.

John Arabin	27 Dec 1755
Sir Daniel Cunninghame	22 Mar. 57

58 Black, Buff Lining, yellow Lace, Am.

Robert Anftruther	28 Dec. 1755

59 Light Crimson, yellow Lace. Ire.

Charles Montagu	30 Dec 1755

60 Royal American, Faced Blue, Am.

E. Loudoun, C Ch	25 Dec 1755
James Abercromby, C.Cn.	2 Dec. 57

John

John Stanwix   1
Joseph Dusseaux   2   } *Jan.* 1756
Charles Jefferyes   3
James Prevost   4
George Aug. Vis. Howe   25 *Feb.* 57
Charles Lawrence   28 *Sept.* 57
Robert Monckton   20 *Dec.* 57

61   Granville Elliott *Brit.*   21 *Apr.* 58
62   William Strode   21 *Apr.* 58
63   David Watson   21 *Apr.* 58
64   Hon. John Barrington   21 *Apr.* 58
65   Robert Armiger   21 *Apr.* 58
66   Edward Sandford   21 *Apr.* 58
67   James Wolfe   21 *Apr.* 58
68   John Lambton   22 *Apr.* 58
69   Hon. Charles Colvill   23 *Apr.* 58
70   John Parslow   27 *Apr.* 58
71   William Petitot   29 *Apr* 58
72   Charles D. of Richmond   9 *May* 58
73   William Browne   30 *Apr.* 58
74   Sharington Talbot   25 *Apr.* 58
75   Hon. John Boscawen   1 *May* 58
76   George Ld. Forbes   22 *Nov.* 56
* 77   Archibald Montgomery   4 *Jan.* 57
* 78   Simon Fraser   5 *Jan.* 57
79   William Draper   2 *Nov.* 57

Rangers in America.

* 80   Thomas Gage   5 *May* 1758

Invalids.

81   Alexander Ld. Lindores   7 *Apr.* 1758
82   John Parker   8 *Apr.* 58

Royal Artillery, Blue faced Red.

Albert Borgard   14 *Apr.* 1705
William Belford   8 *Mar.* 51
Borgard Michelsen   4 *Feb.* 57
* 77, * 78, * 80, *America.*

Master General of ORDNANCE.

1st Colonel Com. ch. R. Regt. Artill.
Note, *l* for Life, *p* for Pleasure.

l. E. of Essex   *Mar.* 29, 1596
p. E. of Devon   *Sept.* 10, 1603
p. E. of Totness   *June* 27, 09
l. Lord Vere   *May* 5, 1617
l. Sir Richard Morrison   *Aug.* 26, 23
l. Sir Thomas Stafford   28
l. E. of Newport   *Sept.* 2, 34
l. Sir William Compton   *Jan.* 22, 60
p. { John Ld Berkeley / John Duncomb, Kt. / Thomas Chicheley } *Oct.* 21 1664
p. Thomas Chicheley, Kt.   4 *Jan.* 1670
p. { Sir John Chicheley / Sir William Hickman / Sir Charles Musgrave } *Jan.* 23 1679
p. Ld Dartmouth   28 *Jan.* 81
p. David Schomberg   28 *Apr.* 89
p. Vis. Sidney   28 *July* 93
p. E. Marlborough   29 *June* 1702
p. Earl Rivers   10 *Jan.* 11
p D. Hamilton   5 *Sept.* 12
p. D. Marlborough   4 *Oct.* 14
p. William E. of Cadogan   30 *June* 22
John D. of Argyll   3 *June* 25
John D. of Montagu   10 *May* 30
Charles D of Marlborough   1755

LIEUT. GENERALS, ib.

Col. en. second and Capt. Cadets.

Sir George Carew   1603
l. Sir William Haydon   35
l. Colin Legg   28 *June* 36
p. David Walter   25 *Nov.* 70
p. George Legg   7 *Dec.* 72
p. Sir Charles Musgrave   28 *Jan.* 81
p Sir Henry Tichbourne   1 *Aug.* 87
p. Sir Henry Goodricke   26 *Apr.* 88
p. John Granville   29 *June* 1702
p. Thomas Erle   2 *May* 05
p. John Hill   21 *June* 12
p. Thomas Erle   20 *Sept.* 14
Thomas Micklethwaite   19 *Mar.* 17
p. Sir Charles Wills   22 *Apr.* 18
p. George Wade F. Marshal   42
p. Sir John Ligonier   48
Lord George Sackville   30 *Nov.* 57

LAND

HORSE GUARDS.

Rank, Colonels.	Lieut. Colonels.	Majors.
1 Lord DeLawarr	{ Gray { Weſt	Bateman Jennings
2 Lord Cadogan	{ Carperter { Deſmarette	Montolieu Sloughter

HORSE GRENADIER GUARDS.

1 Onſlow	Clayton	Bradſhaigh
2 E. of Harrington	Elliot	Mocher

DRAGOON GUARDS.

2 Ld George Sackville	James Muir Campbell	W. Eaſt

DRAGOONS.

1 Hawley	John Toovey	Bartholomew Gallatin
3 E. of Albemarle	Campbell Dalrymple	Francis Bonham
4 Rich, Bt.	Dougla	Brown
7 Cope	George Lawſon Hall	John Litchfield
11 E. of Ancram	Gardner	Warde

FOOT GUARDS.

1 Viſcount Ligonier	Dury	{ Carr { Durand
2 Lord Tyrawly	Noel	{ Julius Cæſar { A'Court
3 E. of Rothes	Robinſon	{ John Griffin Griffin { John Prideaux

FOOT.

3 Howard	Trapaud	Hewett
4 Duroure	Byam Crump	Holly
5 Ld George Bentinck	Irwin	Euſtace
8 Wolfe	Mompeſſon	Cook
11 Bocland	Forreſter	Scott
19 Beauclerck	Douglas	Lumſden
24 Cornwallis	Rufane	Picton
30 E. of Loudoun	Boothby, Bt.	Ramſay
31 Holmes	Lambert	James Vignoles
32 Leighton	M'Dowall	Seton
33 Lord Charles Hay	Ld G. H. Lennox	Daulhat
34 E. of Effingham	Reed .	Dundas
36 Ld Robert Manners	Wilkinſon	Remington
39 Adlercron	Bagſhawe	Francis Forde
_1 Parſons	Weldon	Strode
5_ ____	Wilkinſon	Thomas
56 Ld ____ Manners	Parr	Doyne
6_ E_	Barlow	Teeſdale
62 St_	Jennings	Higginſon
63 Wa__	Deſbriſay	Trollope

Z

64 Bar-

64 Barrington	Pym	Ball
65 Armiger	Salt	Del Garno
66 La Fauffille	Philips	Beauclerck
67 Wolfe	Robinfon	MacDowall
68 Lambton	Adey	Napier
69 Charles Colville	Browne	Martin
70 Parflow	Charles Vignoles	Pigot
71 Petitot	Tayler	Murray
72 D. of Richmond	Carleton	Prefcott
73 William Browne	Fleming	Shirley
74 Sherr. Talbot	Mafters	Maule
75 Bofcawen	Wren	Stuart
79 Eaft-Indies	Diaper	Brereton, Monfon
81 Ld Lindores		Bowles, Brown
82 John Parker		Johnfton, Godfrey

9 Independent Companies.

23 Independent Companies of Invalids.

FORCES in GERMANY.

ROYAL HORSE GUARDS.

Marquis of Granby   James Johnfton   Forbes

DRAGOON GUARDS.

1 Bland	Thomfon	Richardfon
3 Howard	Wade	Fitz Thomas

DRAGOONS.

2 Campbell	Prefton	Blair
6 Cholmondeley	Harvey	Hepburn
10 Mordaunt	Whitley	Sloper

FOOT.

12 Napier	Robinfon	Parry
20 Kingfley	Beckwith	Maxwell
23 Hufke	Pole	Marlay
25 Earl Home	Scott	Goodricke
37 Stuart	Oughton	Hall
51 Brudenell	Buck	Furye

G rife

A. *GIBRALTAR.*

6	Guife	Robert Scott	Williams Bt
7	Ld R bert Bertie	Smith	Gore
13	Pu r cy	Craururd	Chapeau
14	Jefferys	Thomas Lifter	Bell
21	E Po mare	Maxwell	Livingfton
53	Whitmore	A r t	Lindefay
54	John Cary	Renton	Walfh
57	CunynghamcBt	Tow fhend	Onflow

In *A M E R I C A.*

1	ft Wm. 2 Bat	Forfter	Hamilton
15	Amherft	Murray	Farquhar
17	Forbes	Morris	Darby
2	Whitmore	Andrew Ld Rollo	Wrey
27	Ld B akeney	Ha land	Maffey
28	Br gg	Walfh	Dalling
35	Otway	Fletcher	Morris
38	Rofs	Dornellan	Melvill
40	Ho fon	Handfield	Aldridge
42	Ld John Murray	Grant	
43	Kennedy	James	Elliot
44	Abercromby		Eyres
45	Warburton	Wilmot	Murray
46	Murray		Browning
47	Lafcelles	Hale	Huffey
48	Webb	Burton	Rofs
49	Walfh	Spragge	Pepper
55			
58	Anftruther	Howe	Agnew
60	James Abercromby, Commander in Chief.

Stanwix	Bouquet	Robertfon
Prevoft	Haldiman	
Lawrence	Sir John St. Clair Bt.	Prevoft
Monckton	Young	Tullikens
7-} Lt Col.Comdt	{ Montgomery	Grant, Campbell
78 }	{ Frafer	Clephane, Campbell
80	Thomas Gage

I N D E P E N D E N T C O M P A N I E S.

4]		New York.
3	at	S. Carolina.
1		Bermudas.
1]		Providence.

COMPANIES of MARINES.   100 Men each.

Majors, Porfrond, Borcher.
Agent, M. Cuerin, Crown-Court. W. ft z.

Chatham.

Lieutenant Colonel, Bendyfhe.
Majors, Mc. Kenzie, Kempe.
Agent, James Baird, Downing-Str t.

HORSE.

1	John Brown	Charles Ld Moore	Philip Roberts
2	Thomas Bligh	Henry Stamer	Preston
3	Dejean	William Naper	John Rutter
4	H. Seymour Conway	Francis Stuart	Henry Holmes

DRAGOONS.

5	Vt. Molefworth	Clarges	Hill
8	Waldegrave	Severn	Lufhington
9	Honywood	Wynne	Clayton
12	Sir John Whitefoord	Owen	John Wynne
13	Moftyn	Johnfton	John Balaguire
14	Campbell	Eile	Norman

FOOT.

1	St Clair, 1ft Bat.	Horn Elphinfton	Faviere
2	Fitzwilliam	Molefworth	Windus
9	Hon. Jofeph Yorke	Richard Worge	Mufgrave
10	Pole	Gifborne	
16	Handafyd	Laborde	Gabbett
18	Folliott	Armftiong	Hamilton, Bt.
26	Arftiuther	Moncriefi	Erfkine
29	Bofcawen	Richaidfon	Blake
52	Sandford	Mackay	Morgan
59	Montagu	Pitt	Feyrac
76	George Ld Foibes	John Pomeroy	Newton, Chefter,

4 Independent Companies.

ADDITIONS, in IRELAND, 24 Auguft, 1758.

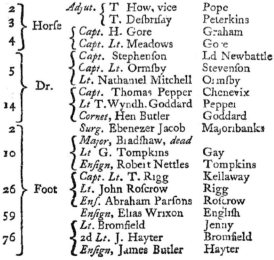

2	Horfe	Adjut. { T How, vice	Pope
3		{ T. Defbrifay	Peterkins
4		{ Capt. H. Gore	Graham
		{ Capt. Lt. Meadows	Go e
5	Dr.	{ Capt. Stephenfon	Ld Newbattle
		{ Capt. Lt. Ormfby	Stevenfon
		{ Lt. Nathaniel Mitchell	Oimfby
14		{ Capt. Thomas Pepper	Chenevix
		{ Lt T.Wyndh. Goddard	Peppei
		{ Cornet, Hen Butler	Goddard
2	Foot	Surg. Ebenezer Jacob	Majoribanks
10		{ Major, Biadfhaw, dead	
		{ Lt G. Tompkins	Gay
		{ Enfign, Robeit Nettles	Tompkins
26		{ Capt. Lt. T. Rigg	Keilaway
		{ Lt. John Rofcrow	Rigg
		{ Enf. Abraham Parfons	Rofcrow
59		Enfign, Elias Wrixon	Englifh
76		{ Lt. Bromfield	Jenny
		{ 2d Lt. J. Hayter	Bromfield
		{ Enfign, James Butler	Hayter

Milton Keynes UK
Ingram Content Group UK Ltd.
UKHW022118231023
431197UK00005B/218